ALSO BY JOSEPH JULIANO, M.D.

When Diabetes Complicates Your Life

The Diabetic's Innovative Cookbook

A Positive Approach to Living with Diabetes

Joseph Juliano, M.D.,
and Dianne Young

HENRY HOLT AND COMPANY
NEW YORK

Henry Holt and Company, Inc.
Publishers since 1866
115 West 18th Street
New York, New York 10011

Henry Holt® is a registered trademark
of Henry Holt and Company, Inc.

Published in Canada by Fitzhenry & Whiteside Ltd.,
195 Allstate Parkway, Markham, Ontario L3R 4T8.

Library of Congress Cataloging-in-Publication Data
Juliano, Joseph.
The diabetic's innovative cookbook: a positive approach to living
with diabetes/Joseph Juliano and Dianne Young.—1st ed.
p.   cm.
Includes bibliographical references and index.
1. Diabetes—Diet therapy.   2. Diabetes—Diet therapy—Recipes.
I. Young, Dianne.   II. Title.
RC662.J85   1994   93-41241
641.5'6314—dc20   CIP

ISBN 0-8050-2518-9
ISBN 0-8050-3785-3 (An Owl Book: pbk.)

Henry Holt books are available for special promotions
and premiums. For details contact: Director, Special Markets.

First published in hardcover in 1994 by
Henry Holt and Company, Inc.

First Owl Book Edition—1995

Designed by Claire Naylon Vaccaro

Printed in the United States of America
All first editions are printed on acid-free paper.∞

1   3   5   7   9   10   8   6   4   2
1   3   5   7   9   10   8   6   4   2
(pbk.)

This book is dedicated to Michael Donahue, without whose keen insight and ability to abstract into and have compassion for the disease diabetes mellitus this book would not have been possible.

— JOSEPH JULIANO

For Frances, who taught me how to cook, and for Wally and Deborah, who made me do it.

— DIANNE YOUNG

Contents

ACKNOWLEDGMENTS
XI

INTRODUCTION
XIII

1. So You Have Diabetes
1

2. The Importance of the Diabetic Diet
6

3. Party Food and Drink
16

4. Restaurant Food
23

5. Holiday Food
28

6. Travel Food
32

7. How About a Late-Night Snack?
38

8. Sweeteners
41

9. Diabetics and Desserts
49

10. A Word About Fiber, Fiber, Fiber
52

11. A Review of the Guidelines for Good Nutrition
66

12. The Importance of Fresh Vegetables and Salads
70

13. Fruit and Fruit Sugar
74

14. Vegetable and Fruit Juices
78

15. *The Role of Family and Friends*
82

16. *Compliance, Diabetes, and a Healthy Life*
87

Introduction to the Recipes
92

Appetizers
95

Breakfast
111

Broths and Soups
125

Sauces, Salsas, Chutneys, and Relishes
161

Salads
183

Vegetables and Side Dishes
213

Rice and Pasta
243

Entrées
261

Desserts
305

EXCHANGE LISTS
365

RAW SHELLFISH WARNING
386

SELECTED READING LIST
388

SUBJECT INDEX
395

RECIPE INDEX
403

Acknowledgments

I would like to gratefully acknowledge Jo Ann, Vic, and Bobby for their relentless hours of assistance in my efforts to write this book. A special acknowledgment goes to Elizabeth Crossman, my editor, who has enabled me to become a better writer.

— JOSEPH JULIANO

I'd like to thank Michael Donahue, my agent, and Elizabeth Crossman, my editor, for all their help and assistance. I'd also like to thank Bobby Macpherson for her inspiration and friendship, as well as Glenn and Cristy, Ricky, Vince, Raymond, Johnny, Mick, Chris, Mickey, Ron, Peggy and Jeff, Kevin T., Alfred, Deb. B., and Bob V., who have encouraged me in my life as well as in my cooking.

— DIANNE YOUNG

Introduction

You are preparing to enter into the pages of an enlightened approach to the diabetic diet. If you are a newly diagnosed diabetic, then you are fortunate indeed to have available a diabetic cookbook that will assist you in better dealing with your diet, a key component of the management strategy of this disease. If you are a long-term diabetic, then I feel sure you will agree that this book is unlike any others on the market today.

While not intended to be a medical text or technical treatise on the diabetic diet, this book does contain the information necessary to the understanding of the importance of diet therapy within the total diabetes management program. You will find that the all too familiar restrictions within the diabetic diet are played down, as the commitment of this book is to the positive attitudinal approach of what *can* be done rather than what cannot be done. In my opinion, the opinion of a person who has lived with the disease for three decades, it is time we approached chronic diseases and the progressive complications they can entail with the most positive mind-set humanly possible. This, I feel, will set up long-range reference points that hopefully will greatly benefit the day-to-day condition and diminish negative expectations.

If you are told over and over again that you are going to suffer terribly in trying to cope with your diabetes and manage your dietary restrictions, the reference points will soon be set up in your mind to enable the condition to affect you with its full power. If, on the other hand, your mental reference points are set up to accept only the most positive information, then, should the worst things begin to manifest themselves, the positive person will be better equipped to fight off these complications and thus achieve a better quality of life. I feel that this is important in all aspects of life, so why should we not approach the nature of the diabetic diet in a similar positive manner?

I do not want to make you feel for even one second that this cookbook is based on fantasy and that this positive thinking is only for a bunch of kooks who eat seaweed and meditate on top of a mountain somewhere in Tibet. Personally, I have enlisted positive mind-sets to overcome extreme adversity in living with diabetes. As I write these words, I am into my thirtieth year with Type I diabetes, or insulin-dependent diabetes mellitus, also known as juvenile-onset diabetes. Seven years ago, I suffered one of the more devastating complications of diabetes, total blindness, after having twenty-fifteen — better than normal — vision all my life. You see, I truly know what it means to utilize positive thinking in order to save one's life. Perhaps this is a new approach for you. If it is, you may require a great deal of mental reprogramming to rid yourself of many years of negative expectations. If you are already a positive-thinking person, then this book will easily fit into your repertoire of tools needed to better cope with diabetes.

This book is the result of a team effort to produce the finest diabetic cookbook on the market today. Certainly, it cannot be all things to all diabetics. However, every recipe was created and tested by a gourmet chef and scrutinized for the exchanges within the diabetic meal plan by a registered dietitian with an expertise in diabetes. Because some of these recipes may tend to be rather avant-garde, it is up to you to monitor your caloric intake so that you do not become overweight or hyperglycemic. Good diabetes management practice is mandatory and is implied at all times, but only you can balance and manage your dietary intake properly. This book will provide you with an alternative to the rather drab clinical thinking that was so prevalent in the past. If we stir your thinking and gastronomical delight to a state of high excitement, then we have indeed done our job well.

Cheers and *bon appétit!*

1

So You Have Diabetes

You look down at your solid gold Rolex and realize that it is time to leave to pick up your dinner companion. As you turn the sterling silver ignition key of your Ferrari F40 street-legal race car, the roar of the fuel-injected twelve cylinders, four cams, and forty-eight valves makes it a little difficult to hear your dinner date's voice on the cellular phone. You pull into the driveway; your dinner date is immaculately dressed and looks fantastic. So now, it's off to the finest restaurant in town for a late-night dinner. As you pull up to the restaurant, you notice that everyone must be driving a Cadillac, Mercedes, or Porsche these days. The oil tycoons that usually have dinner at this restaurant are here in force tonight.

Once inside and seated, you peruse the menu and place your order with the elegantly attired waiter: "We will start with a bowl of New England clam chowder and garlic bread. Then, the rib eye, extra-large cut, cooked in butter, and rare. Baked potato with butter, sour cream, and chives, the broccoli with Béarnaise sauce, and blue cheese dressing on the salad. And we will both have a double vodka martini, shaken, not stirred.

"And, waiter, prepare the Dutch Chocolate Fudge Royale 'Death by Chocolate' Flambé for two as our dessert selection."

Wow, this must be some kind of dream! I mean, who can afford to eat like this today? Even if you can afford it financially, affording it in terms of your health could be quite expensive indeed, especially if this were done often. Well, you have got one thing right, it is a dream. In fact, for most of us diabetics, the above scenario can be a wonderful fantasy, and, like most fantasies, should be kept that way. But I think you can still eat well-balanced gourmet meals without the fat-intensive, high-protein load described above, and in this book I will show you how it can be done.

So you have diabetes. Well, welcome to the club. Unfortunately, the diabetes club is really not an exclusive club at all. There are approximately fifteen million of us today who have been diagnosed with diabetes mellitus, the majority of that number being Type II non-insulin-dependent diabetics. There may well be another fifteen million undiagnosed diabetics, who have either Type I diabetes, insulin-dependent diabetes mellitus (IDDM) or Type II, non-insulin-dependent diabetes mellitus (NIDDM), and do not know it.

Back to the fantasy scene for just a minute. Have you ever noticed how fanatic the owners of some types of cars can be? Never, but never, would they entertain the thought of putting anything but the best gasoline and oil into their cars for the most efficient and highest performance of their engines. And how about the owners of Learjets or Cessna Citations? Do you think they would put some sort of watered down aviation fuel into those babies? No way, only the best.

But when it comes to the finest machines on the face of the earth, our bodies, many of us do not think much about the quality of fuel we put into them. A friend of mine, a former physician to the NASA astronauts, related this story concerning this country's highly qualified, highly educated, and top physically conditioned test pilots, the NASA astronauts. As their physician, he was able to fly with them in their training jet, the T-38. After one mission from Houston to El Paso, the doctor and the astronaut he had accompanied went into the flight center. The astronaut went over to a vending machine and got a soda and a sticky-sweet honey bun for his lunch. The T-38 jet was being fueled with the finest JP-24 aviation jet fuel, while the astronaut was refueling with garbage. Now this is really an interesting phenomenon. How long can we do things like this to our bodies and expect them to run at maximum efficiency and peak performance levels? Can we go out late at night and eat a high-fat meal and expect to feel good the next day?

Now that you have decided to take steps in dealing with your diabetes — to eat the correct foods for a demanding, progressive disease that is here for the duration of your life, at least until some sort of miraculous cure can be found — you will find that educating yourself in terms of nutrition will be greatly rewarding for you.

The fact that you have diabetes requires an adjustment in your lifestyle, daily routine, and habits. A definite positive mind-set to a more healthy lifestyle is in your best interest, and eating the right things and in the right amounts will take some getting used to. It is really not all that difficult. In fact, when you get down to the bottom line, it is all a matter of proper education and common sense.

For instance, consider our earlier fantasy scene. Is it really a good idea to have a fat-laced steak late at night? It has been proven scientifically that eating a meal that is high in calories, and especially high in fats and protein, causes internal organs such as the kidneys, liver, and heart to work much harder in their efforts to process this intensive meal. We know that this is not good for us, and for the diabetic, eating such a heavy meal late in the evening means throwing off our schedule.

My point is that in order to obtain the best control of diabetes, it is important to maintain normal mealtimes and make this a part of your diabetic management routine. In the case of the insulin-dependent diabetic, if the evening insulin injection is normally taken at six P.M., the evening meal should follow within thirty minutes. Taking the insulin injection at six P.M. and waiting until nine P.M. to eat the evening meal is not acceptable due to the possible rapid fall in blood glucose that may occur after the insulin injection is taken. The diabetic will learn how important keeping a routine schedule is when it comes to mealtimes. I think some latitude can be given, but, generally, most doctors and dietitians advise that diabetics' meals be timed within thirty minutes of administration of the insulin injection or of taking oral antidiabetic medication. Guidelines for the scheduling of your insulin injections and mealtimes should be carefully discussed with your doctor, as this is a very important aspect within the diabetic management program.

I am sure that you are aware that the disease diabetes mellitus is an overwhelmingly complex set of diseases within a disease. Because everyone with diabetes is an individual case, what is good for you and your case of diabetes may not be exactly right for me or another person with diabetes. This book can give only the basic guidelines that have worked well for me during my thirty years of living with this complicated disease. You absolutely must — and I will say this over and over again throughout this book — discuss all aspects of your diabetes with your own personal health management team. This is vitally important in all areas of therapy for diabetes, and the diabetic diet is one of these areas. Becoming an expert in the management of your diabetic diet will lead to your becoming an expert in all areas of diabetes management.

Okay, let's now take a deep breath and explore briefly in the following chapters some of the various aspects of the diabetic diet. Through the use of management and nutritional information from the American Diabetes Association, the American Dietetic Association, the American Heart Association, the National Cancer Institute, and anecdotes based on my personal experience, you will learn some basic guidelines and develop strategies that will help you live with your diabetes and the diabetic diet on a daily basis. Again, you will want to take on the most positive mind-set and open up the opportunities for better nutrition, thus leading to a healthier lifestyle.

The Importance of the Diabetic Diet

The American Diabetes Association Diabetic Exchange Lists (see pages 365–85) were developed jointly by the American Diabetes Association and the American Dietetic Association and actually form the backbone of the diabetic diet.

These exchange lists, wherein one food can be substituted for another based on the breakdown of the foods in terms of carbohydrates, fats, protein, and sugar, were first developed in the early sixties. They were revised in 1986. It is from these lists that your individual diet can be tailored to your activity level or the amount of exercise you do, the amount of insulin or oral antidiabetic medication you take, your age group, your own specific caloric requirements, and your own particular lifestyle. As you become more familiar with the exchange lists, you will develop a better understanding of the manipulations that are possible. This understanding will help you to manage your new diet, but it will require time, study, patience, and a good positive attitude.

Let me recall for you my own feelings when as a teenager I first heard about my new diabetic diet. One of the grinding dilemmas that confronted my family and me when I was first diagnosed was the emotional overload of being told I would have to be on a diet for the rest of my life. And not just any diet, but a very special intake-restricted diet that would be an integral part of the therapy designed to prolong my life. Think about this for just a minute. The word *diet* has all the connotations that make most people cringe with dread. When told that this diet will restrict you from many of the items that make a meal at the very least appetizing and appealing, the cringing and the dread turn into fear and depression.

The diabetic manuals of thirty years ago listed columns of re-stricted food. I would play games with these lists and recite the long columns of restricted items. My family would just look at me and wonder what it was exactly that I could eat. Of course, everything with sugar was either restricted entirely or limited to minute quan-tities. After some time contemplating the diabetic diet, my mother figured that I could eat green beans, onions, lettuce, cucumbers, and other vegetables containing no calories in unlimited quantities. It is no wonder that even today I am a voracious salad eater, never having tired of a wonderful tossed salad with a myriad of garden vegetables. But oh boy, guess what? It seemed I had these unrestricted items at every meal. Even while I was in the hospital getting adjusted to my insulin requirements, one of the staples at lunch and dinner was an onion salad. This onion salad consisted of sliced onions and vinegar. That's right, no oil or salad dressing was added to this delicious little salad and even today, I break out in a cold sweat when I think of an onion salad with just vinegar as the salad dressing. In fact, violent thoughts enter my mind.

All kidding aside, the hospital food-service staff tried their best to serve me decent meals during my stay. For breakfast, there were powdered eggs cooked without even a hint of butter, limp white-bread toast with a drop of margarine, skim milk that was so watery it was blue in color, and if I was lucky, a strip or two of bacon that had been sacrificed to the fire gods. I know, you think I am still kidding, but actually I am serious. You see, the meals for diabetics were not too creative in those days. But here is the important thing to consider: even thirty years ago, dietitians and nutritionists knew that foods high in fat and sugar were not good for the diabetic.

But what about all the rest of the people out there? I must admit that even at fifteen I seriously wondered how it would be if everyone had to be on a diabetic diet just like mine. Now take a look at nutritionists' most recent dietary recommendations for Americans. They look suspiciously similar to the new diabetic diet of today. Over the years, I have often wondered what the general health of the average American would be like if over twenty-five years ago everyone had been placed on a diabetic diet. Would we still be seeing the overabundance of clogged arteries, coronary artery disease, arteriosclerosis, and stroke that we see today? Would our children be better informed of the potential danger of ingesting cereals sweetened with indecently high levels of refined sugar? Would the general population be more trim, less lethargic, and less overweight?

Certainly, I cannot answer these questions; however, I have often regarded the diabetic diet as a very healthful diet. It is very interesting indeed that diets recommended by the American Heart Association and the American Cancer Society closely resemble today's diabetic diet. Fortunately, we have seen the diabetic diet improve with the advancement of food science, and this science is reflected in the high technology used in modern food chemistry and processing.

When I think back to my initial days with my new diabetic diet, the onion salads and the bland, tasteless, colorless, and odorless preparations, I try not to become emotionally involved again, but to remember those days with a little humor and marvel at how far we have advanced. Let's look at the positive side of being on a lifelong diabetic diet. Today the backbone of the diabetic meal-planning philosophy remains the careful management of food and caloric quantity, avoidance of refined sugar, lowered fat intake, and now most important, restricted protein intake. Later we will talk more about the reasons why a restricted amount of protein may be very beneficial to the diabetic.

In any diabetic management program, there are key words you must remember. For the Type I insulin-dependent diabetic, these words are *insulin, diet,* and *exercise.* For the Type II non-insulin-dependent diabetic, the words are *oral antidiabetic medication, diet,* and *exercise.* In either case, diet plays a crucial role in the management therapy regime. In fact, if you are non-insulin-dependent, diet can be so crucial that if it is carefully managed, your diabetes may become less severe and the possibility exists that your diabetes may diminish altogether.

However, if this is to occur, it will require tremendous determination and discipline on your part. Typically, a non-insulin-dependent diabetic will begin a diet with a valiant effort at first, then the tendency to pick up old eating habits becomes greater and greater. This of course includes eating sweet foods such as pies, cakes, and cookies, which a diabetic should closely watch. If additional weight is gained, oral medication must be increased due to higher blood sugar values, thus creating a vicious cycle. It would seem that the reward of diminished severity of diabetes would keep a person from eating the wrong items and from overeating in general, but unfortunately, this is not always the case.

A question I often ask myself is, If I were given the choice of never having to give myself another insulin injection, would I be willing to be so disciplined in managing my diet, exercise, and body weight that I'd risk becoming fanatic about my diabetes management? This would be a very difficult question to answer. Many Type II non-insulin-dependent diabetics face the same dilemma, but from a slightly different angle. You see, I am already on insulin therapy and have been for nearly thirty years. The question I posed for myself is purely theoretical. But, for the Type II diabetic who is not presently on injectable insulin therapy, the question often becomes a real one, as illustrated below.

After a routine physical examination and blood chemistry, Mr. Jones's doctor has some startling news: "Mr. Jones, you are over-weight and have a fasting blood sugar of over three hundred and fifty. Your triglycerides are elevated and your total cholesterol is high at two hundred and seventy-five. Your HDL cholesterol, the good guys, is low. Your LDL cholesterol, the bad guys, is high. We will begin you immediately on a diabetic diet, which will be a very restricted calorie, high-carbohydrate, low-protein diet that will also be high in dietary fiber in order to lower your triglycerides and cholesterol. We will also begin you on an oral antidiabetic medication that will help your pancreas deliver insulin and thus lower your blood sugar. Now, do you have any questions?"

Dumbfounded, Mr. Jones can barely think straight, much less formulate one of the hundreds of questions that are reeling in his mind. However, once he accepts and better understands his condition as a newly diagnosed Type II diabetic, the following question will most likely be asked of him: "Do you think you have the willpower, discipline, and tenacity to watch your diet so strictly and manage your caloric intake with adequate exercise so as to reduce your oral anti-diabetic medication to the point that you no longer require it and then to lose your excess weight and possibly reverse your diabetic condition?" This is a very big question and for many it is just not possible. But for those with the will and discipline, it could mean a great deal.

For those of us who are insulin-dependent, with strict dietary management, exercise, and careful regulation of our blood sugar and insulin intake we too can benefit in terms of lowering our insulin requirements and maintaining less body fat, thus hopefully preventing or delaying the onset of long-term complications.

It is best for you to understand from the outset that diabetics, both Type I insulin-dependent diabetics and Type II non-insulin-dependent diabetics, are prone to long-term complications that are rather unique to the diabetic condition. It is therefore vitally important that you manage your disease with the utmost level of control. I will not delve into diabetic complications in this book except in general terms. There are many good works available on the subject of diabetic complications and you should study them (see the Selected Reading List, pp. 388–94) and consult frequently with your doctor and health management team. Diabetes requires a commitment to careful management over the long term — not for just today or tomorrow, but for the rest of your life.

A More Technical Discussion

I would now like to enter into a more technical discussion regarding the diabetic diet and the position that is currently held by the American Diabetes Association regarding the best research into the health and nutritional requirements necessary for the diabetic.

A position statement by the American Diabetes Association is formulated at intervals when research into the nutritional requirements of diabetics so warrants. A report first published in 1979, entitled "Principles of Nutrition and Dietary Guidelines for Individuals with Diabetes Mellitus," was a joint effort of the Food and Nutrition committees of the American Diabetes Association. This report was published due to the new data found through research and improved methodology of the factors involved with the diabetic diet and blood glucose. In March 1991, a medical report appearing in *Diabetes Care*, volume 14, supplement 2, contained important information regarding the position taken by the American Diabetes Association. This article, entitled "Nutritional Recommendations and

Principles for Individuals with Diabetes Mellitus," is an overview of the recommendations for good nutrition and better health for the diabetic population. Both reports emphasize good diabetes management and blood glucose control in combination with changes in the blood lipid levels, reflecting the increased awareness of fat in our diets and the increased research into the field of lipid biochemistry.

Since the publication of the 1979 report, a vast amount of new data has been collected in the field of nutrition and the management of diabetes. Many new ideas have come to light in view of the questions arising from (1) the optimal carbohydrate, protein, and fat intake, (2) the role of fiber, (3) the role of the glycemic index and its relationship to food exchanges, and (4) the role of eicosapentanoic acid or fish oil. By the 1980s, a transformation occurred and many advances were made in nutrition education.

It is now well established that nutritional recommendations for diabetics closely resemble those of the American Heart Association, the National Cancer Institute, the Nutritional Committee for Recommendations for Children with Diabetes of the American Academy of Pediatrics, and the 1985 U.S. Dietary Guidelines.

These nutritional recommendations are as follows:

1. Caloric Intake

Calories should be prescribed to achieve and maintain a desirable body weight.

2. Carbohydrate Intake

a. The amount of carbohydrates should be liberalized, ideally 50 percent to 60 percent of the total calories, and individualized with the amount dependent on the impact on blood glucose and lipid levels and individual eating patterns.

b. Whenever acceptable to the patient, foods containing un-refined carbohydrates with fiber should be substituted for highly refined carbohydrates, which are low in fiber.

c. In some individuals, modest amounts of sucrose and other refined sugars may be acceptable contingent on metabolic control and body weight.

3. Protein Intake

It is now generally recognized that Americans consume too much protein. The recommended dietary allowance for protein is 0.8 grams per kilogram of body weight for adults. Elderly people may require more than the recommended daily allowance (RDA). There are circumstances where the protein intake may need to be reduced, for example, in patients with incipient renal disease.

4. Total Fat and Cholesterol Intake

Total fat and cholesterol intake should be restricted. Total fat should make up less than 30 percent of total calories and cholesterol should be limited to less than 300 milligrams per day. This level of intake may be difficult, but it is a goal worth attaining. Replacement of saturated fat with unsaturated fat may slow the progression of atherosclerosis, clogged arteries. The addition of certain fats, such as eicosapentanoic acid, fish oil, and monounsaturated fats, may be acceptable; however, more research is needed to define their value.

5. Alternative Sweeteners

The use of various nutritive and nonnutritive sweeteners is acceptable in the management of diabetes.

6. Salt Intake

Many Americans eat more salt than is advisable. The recommended sodium intake is 1,000 milligrams per 100 kilocalories, not to exceed 300 milligrams per day. In hypertensive subjects, salt may be harmful and therefore intake should be reduced. Severe sodium restriction could also be harmful for certain individuals with poorly controlled diabetes, postural hypotension, and fluid imbalance.

7. Alcohol

The same precautions regarding alcohol that apply to the general public apply to people with diabetes. Specific problems may occur with hypoglycemia (low blood sugar), neuropathy (nerve damage), glycemic control, obesity, and/or hyperlipidemia. Please see my discussion of alcohol and diabetics in the next chapter.

8. Vitamins and Minerals

Vitamins and minerals should meet the recommended requirements for health. There is no evidence unique to the patient with diabetes to warrant supplementation of vitamin and mineral intake unless the patient is on a very low calorie diet or other special circumstances exist. Calcium supplements may be necessary under special circumstances.

9. Goals for Diabetes Management

a. Restore normal blood glucose and optimal lipid levels. Maintain blood glucose as near to physiological as possible to (1) prevent hyperglycemia (high blood sugar) and/or hypoglycemia (low blood sugar); (2) prevent or delay long-term cardiovascular, renal, retinal, or neurological complications associated with diabetes mellitus; and (3) contribute to a normal outcome of pregnancy for women with diabetes.

b. Maintain normal growth rate in children and adolescents and attain and maintain reasonable body weight in adolescents and adults. Any abnormal unexplained deviation in growth rate or weight gain or loss as plotted on standard grids warrants an assessment of diabetes control, eating behavior, and caloric intake in consideration of alternative problems or diagnosis.

c. Provide adequate nutrition for the pregnant woman, the fetus, and lactation.

d. Stay consistent in the timing of meals and snacks to prevent inordinate swings in blood glucose levels for people using exogenous insulin.

e. Determine a meal plan appropriate for the individual's lifestyle based on a diet history. Blood glucose monitoring results can then be used to integrate insulin therapy with the usual as well as unacceptable eating and exercise patterns.

10. Weight Management

Weight management for obese people with non-insulin-dependent diabetes mellitus involves specific changes in food intake and eating behavior as well as increased activity levels. Continued support and follow-up by qualified professionals are important if long-term lifestyle changes are to be made.

3

Party Food and Drink

The Adult Party

*E*very so often, the cocktail party comes around, and every now and then it is a social requirement that you attend. But what about your diabetes? Of course, as a diabetic, you should carefully monitor how much alcohol you drink and also carefully scrutinize each and every wonderfully rich, fatty, salty, high-calorie hors d'oeuvre. Is there a party rationale you can adopt so that the party can be enjoyed and guilt feelings and high blood sugar do not completely ruin everything?

Yes, I think we can develop a strategy that will enable you to attend these functions and better prepare you for the adjustment in both your dietary requirements and the schedule you normally maintain. With a few simple pointers, I think you will feel more at ease in attending these functions and will not dread their inevitability.

In most adult situations, a cocktail party means alcoholic beverages will be served. Drinking as a diabetic is a dangerous proposition for many reasons, but I feel it should be your personal choice. Many diabetics choose to drink some form of alcohol, but in my opinion, mixing alcohol and diabetes is a risky business. You must consult with your doctor and dietitian concerning this aspect of the diabetic diet.

There are several aspects of alcohol that make it dangerous for the diabetic. First, the sugar content of alcoholic beverages is quite high. This is true of beer and wine as well as distilled whiskey, vodka, bourbon, tequila, and many others. Scotch seems to have less sugar than most other whiskeys. There are some exchanges that may be given up to account for a glass of beer or wine, but excess in this area should be carefully avoided.

Also, alcohol does have a blood sugar–lowering effect and can numb the senses that help provide clues to your physical state as a diabetic after you have ingested alcohol. Even when consumed in moderate amounts, alcohol dulls the senses and impairs judgment. So, for instance, if you were to go to a cocktail party, eat some of the hors d'oeuvres, and drink three or four Scotch whiskeys, you might then return home and fall asleep on the sofa. If you were then to have an insulin reaction or hypoglycemia, the alcoholic effect might so numb your senses that the insulin reaction's symptoms would go unnoticed. If you continued to remain asleep and the insulin reaction continued untreated, you could fall into a diabetic hypoglycemic coma. This seems to be the manner in which many diabetics have passed away. For these diabetics, the combination of alcohol and an insulin reaction proved fatal. I am not saying that this will happen in every instance; however, you should be acutely aware of this possibility when you consider drinking alcohol and living with diabetes. Remember, an insulin reaction is life-threatening and could mean coma and death if it is not treated with a source of glucose.

The other pitfall for diabetics is the appetizers served at cocktail parties. Dips and chips, Swedish meatballs, rich cheeses, sliced cold cuts, fried foods, and many other favorite hors d'oeuvre selections at cocktail parties usually are not intended for the person who is diet conscious and should not replace a main meal. The diabetic must be cautious in two respects: not to gorge on the great-tasting appetizers and not to skip a normal meal by eating appetizers that do not make up a full meal's worth of calories.

Prepare a plan of action and have ready easy responses to those who may try to entice you to drink or eat more than you should. My general rule of thumb is to eat a light meal before I go and to drink some fruit juice and a large glass of water. In this way, I can take my insulin injection knowing I will have adequate calories working for me so that I do not fall into an insulin reaction. Also, because I have taken the edge off my appetite, I will not gorge on the hors d'oeuvres.

Set a definite limit on the quantity of alcohol you will consume and remain disciplined and adamant about this imposed limit. Have in mind the types of appetizers that you will allow yourself to enjoy and set a limit on quantity. When I attend a cocktail party, I let myself taste several selections of appetizers. By allowing myself to selectively sample, I feel as though I am not restricting myself too greatly and am part of the crowd. This strategy has worked for me and I have even been able to keep some semblance of normal blood sugar after the party.

I will admit, however, that developing this strategy did not occur overnight. I have many years of experience living with diabetes and have learned some tricks along the way. It is some of these valuable experiences of "living with diabetes on a daily basis" that I want to share with you.

When I was younger, I went to parties without knowing how to deal with the food and alcohol. If you simply let yourself go, then you may either eat too much, eat too little, or consume too much alcohol. After all, it is easier to get into the party spirit after a couple of drinks. It is my opinion that with some planning and strategy — keeping your own best interests in mind in dealing with your diabetes — you can attend the party and enjoy it as much or even more than the others.

And don't forget that today many wise hosts prepare a tray of fresh sliced raw vegetables that can make great appetizers for the diabetic, and with some dip or salad dressing, can be a wonderful substitute for chips. My final word of advice here is not to be too hard on yourself while not allowing yourself to get out of control, either. Balance in all things is my motto.

The Young Person's Party

"Hey, Joe, this is John. What's going on, space cadet?"

"Hey, what's happening, John?"

"Well, my mom is planning my birthday party this Friday and we want you and Paul to come over. My dad's going to barbeque hamburgers and hot dogs and then we're going to pig out on birthday cake. I guess they really want to celebrate my fifteenth birthday. Can you make it? It's gonna be awesome!"

"Oh, man, John. I don't know."

"What do you mean, you don't know, dude? We are talking free food and a party here."

"Yeah, yeah, I know. But it's my diabetes. I don't think I can eat any of the stuff you are talking about."

"What? Hey, wow, earth to Joe. What do you mean diabetes, anyway? When did you get that? Are you sick or something?"

"Naw, man, I'm not sick or anything. It's just that I don't know if I can eat the things you are talking about at your party. You know, the cake and stuff."

"Gosh, Joe, now you're gonna tell me you can't eat cake or cookies anymore, right?"

"Pretty much. I am restricted from eating cake, cookies, and anything with lots of sugar in it. I don't know how to juggle my diet to handle the party deal, man."

"Oh, come on, dude. If we don't have you at the party, it's gonna be nowhere. You've just gotta come and party with me, Joe."

"All right. My parents and I will look at my diabetic meal plan to see how I can rearrange my schedule. But you know I can only drink diet colas and sodas without sugar now, don't you?"

"Yeah, I thought you were turning into some sort of health freak when I saw you drinking diet colas and eating salads in the school cafeteria. Now I understand, man. You're gonna have to teach me about diabetes. I really don't know anything about it at all, except my uncle died from it, I think."

And so it goes. Another teenager is pressed into admission of his newly acquired disease and forced to deal with it. How can Joe go to the party and eat what the others eat and yet still maintain his diet on the diabetic meal plan?

Let's take a closer look at the typical party situation. If this is Joe's first party after his diagnosis of diabetes, then some planning is necessary. This requires a conference with Mom and Dad or with Joe's doctor or dietitian, in order to set up a strategy.

Now let's consider the birthday party menu. If the party goers are having hamburgers and hot dogs prepared on the barbeque, there will be no problem with these food items. A lean hamburger, well cooked and drained of any grease, especially cooked on the outside barbeque, along with mustard and a slice of low-fat cheese is a good meal. If the bun is whole wheat, and lettuce, tomato, dill pickle, and onion are added (none of which contain sugar and therefore add no significant calories to the diabetic meal), it is even better. Catsup and other sweet sauces contain a tremendous amount of sugar and should always be avoided. Mayonnaise can be substituted for mustard, but remember, this is a fat exchange, and since this party food is already fat intensive, mustard would be the better choice.

There will probably be potato chips at the party, and unfortunately, eating a potato chip is just about as inadvisable as eating a teaspoon of sugar, due to the tremendous amount of fat and oil in their processing. But who can avoid the chips, especially a teenager who if given a choice would probably live on a diet of various chips alone? I would suggest some talk about this part of the diet because we all have a weakness for those chips, which seem to go so well with a party. Many people are more aware of the high fat content of chips today and serve raw vegetables and dip along with chips. Dips can also be high in fats, so caution must be exercised here as well, but the vegetables are an excellent alternative for a diabetic. If the teen insists on chips, then perhaps placing a small amount on the plate as a chip allowance would work, keeping in mind the discipline necessary to prevent overeating of chips and the resulting high blood sugar.

Teens and most everyone else here on earth enjoy cake or some form of dessert on a birthday. Along with the cake is some form of drink, usually sugar sodas or other sugar drinks that a diabetic cannot have. Still, this shouldn't prevent Joe from attending the party.

How about calling John's parents and giving them a talk about diabetes in plain language? If John's uncle had diabetes, then surely John's parents will be only too understanding. And I think you will find this to be true as you explain diabetes to most people today. Explain that Joe can no longer drink sugar soft drinks. Natural fruit drinks such as pure orange juice and apple juice are great, but these juices contain a large quantity of natural fruit sugar (fructose), which will cause Joe's blood sugar to skyrocket if he has just an eight-ounce glass. Fruit juice could be given in controlled amounts as a fruit exchange, however, and worked out for this meal if Joe so chooses. Ask if it would be possible to have a few sugarless soft drinks at the party. If it isn't, then Joe could take a few of his own favorites to the party. Problem number one solved.

Now, what about the cake? Well, what about it? You know it contains a lot of sugar. Almost all cakes do. In fact, most cakes contain at least two cups of sugar or more in their initial ingredients list. And this is not to mention the icing, which is usually composed entirely of butter and sugar. The icing can simply be scraped off the cake, and if Joe does not eat a huge piece, then he can enjoy a piece of cake, without icing, like the rest of his friends.

This is the new attitude that must come into play when Joe is at any social gathering where the meals will be different. The diabetic child will be faced with eating and dietary challenges for the duration of his or her life. Indeed, the diabetic diet must be thought of as a discipline forever, not just for today. I believe that a totally restrictive attitude should be avoided. The positive attitude of taking a close look at what can be done, rather than what cannot be done, is the future for all new diabetic attitudinal thinking whether it concerns diet or not. Again, we want to stress to the diabetic child the importance of balance, moderation, and healthy food intake, which will greatly benefit not only the diabetic child but also the entire family.

4

Restaurant Food

hat fantastic restaurant choices we have today — fast-food restaurants, hamburger stands, cafés, diners, and white-tablecloth restaurants. There is an absolutely amazing number of restaurants to choose from, representing a tremendous variety of cuisines: Mexican, Greek, Italian, Chinese, Ethiopian, and Vietnamese, to name just a few.

As diabetics, we must consider what we need to do so that we too can enjoy the convenience, social activity, and pure enjoyment of eating out. Again, a strategy and mind-set must be developed for one's own individual case of diabetes and eating preferences. And the demands of the diabetic diet regime must be factored into the equation. At times this can be a difficult task, especially for the inexperienced diabetic.

I had been diagnosed as a diabetic only six months earlier when my best friend's family asked me to accompany them for dinner at one of Washington, D.C.'s finest French restaurants. I wanted to go very badly, but how would I manage the rich French cuisine with its wine and butter sauces? After all, this kind of food was not allowed for on my diabetic exchange list. How was I to compute my caloric intake for my diet? I will never forget how nervous I was at the restaurant, because at that time my mother was in complete control of my dietary intake. At this early stage of the game, I even came home from school at lunchtime in order to strictly control my diet, rather than eat at the school cafeteria. When my best friend asked me what dessert I wanted after our terrific French meal, I replied that I could not eat any sweet desserts. He immediately frowned, so I retorted with "Well, wait till you get diabetes someday." His older brother was sitting next to us, and I distinctly remember how he got a big smile on his face and laughed at my statement.

A lot of experience and time have come and gone since then. After the first year with diabetes, I decided that eating at the school cafeteria with my friends would be better than going home to eat. An active high-school social life required that I learn to balance my diet for both dating and other school activities where eating was the main event. Because I was well educated in my dietary requirements through the efforts of my mother and father, I became at ease as the transition was made through high school and into college. Actually, I became a health nut, going to the local health food store and eating a large amount of fresh vegetables and salads. As you gain experience with the food exchanges and approximate quantities, you will develop a keen sense of which foods you can eat and which you should avoid when you eat out.

As a basic beginning psychology when going out to eat at a restaurant, give yourself the freedom of having anything on the menu. This freedom will allow you to make choices just as any nondiabetic person would at the restaurant. Does this mean you should choose the selection with the highest sugar and fat content on the menu? Would you normally choose this selection if you did not have diabetes, or is this selection made in protest of the fact that you are now a diabetic? If you crave an item that is a poor choice for you or if you simply are protesting, to what lengths should you go to stop yourself from indulging?

This is a judgment call that you will have to make. If your mind insists, then go ahead and have the selection. The key factor here is not to eat as much of this particular selection as you would another less calorie-intensive selection. In this manner, you will not feel deprived, and with some discipline and good management, you too can enjoy almost any selection that any menu has to offer. Quantity is the key factor.

We will discuss this psychology again in dealing with sweets and desserts. Of course, there are selections on any given menu that are more preferable and less preferable or even inappropriate for one with diabetes. For a person with my level of experience in living with diabetes, it is very clear to me what selections I should seriously consider on any restaurant menu. For those of you who are newly diagnosed, or who have never had the requirement of watching your dietary intake before, the process will be a little more difficult at first.

The first thing I am interested in knowing about on a menu is the salads. I usually have a salad with my dinner meal, and I will often have a salad for lunch. I can make an entire meal of a chef's salad or some type of interesting seafood salad. But what if you do not like salads? The American Heart Association and the National Cancer Institute advise eating fresh leafy vegetables on a daily basis, and the inclusion of fresh vegetables within the diabetic meal plan is vitally important. If you are a meat-and-potatoes type who has never liked salads, can you train yourself to eat more vegetables and salads as if they were medicine? I know this is a tough requirement for those who do not like vegetables in any form or fashion; however, it would certainly be in your best interest to develop a taste for salads and fresh vegetables.

After I decide what salad I am going to have, I then make a choice for the main selection. Ninety-nine percent of the time, I do not even consider any fried foods, even though I know fried food tastes great. I still eat Kentucky Fried Chicken occasionally, but I do not eat a lot of it and I try to keep that treat to a minimum. We all know what happens when we diabetics have too much of a good thing: high blood sugar and excessive weight gain. Today even the fast-food restaurants are aware that most Americans should restrict their intake of saturated fats and fried foods, so there is usually a broiled or baked selection that will be more appropriate for the diabetic.

If your favorite order is a double-bacon, double-cheese, double-meat sourdough burger with everything on it, large fries, extra catsup, and a large Diet Coke, you are going to ingest a large quantity of fat, salt, protein, and sugar. I realize that this type of burger is the ultimate choice for taste; however, it is really not a very good choice in terms of health. Perhaps once in a while you can splurge on some fast food in this manner, but not often.

There are two problems here. First, the fries are cooked in, and usually drenched with, oil. This means more fat added to your diet. Second, the tomato catsup has a high sugar and salt content. What I am saying here is to carefully monitor these items and watch the quantity you eat. In the sixties, these items were simply forbidden on the diabetic meal plan. I think I consumed my share of catsup anyway, but I suffered in terms of high blood sugar. At least today we have the ability to test our blood sugar and determine the level of high or low blood sugar we are experiencing. Our control level, for the average diabetic who desires to well control his or her disease, is dramatically increased.

Better choices for the diabetic are any of the less fat-intensive items. Fast-food restaurants usually have a breakdown chart available describing the various quantities of carbohydrates, proteins, and fats along with the amount of sodium or salt found in their meals. If you have a favorite fast-food restaurant, look over the chart and try to determine if your favorite selection is appropriate for your meal planning. Thankfully, many of these restaurants are putting in salad bars or selections such as chicken salads or taco salads that make a nice choice for the diabetic.

I do not want to belabor the point of the care the diabetic needs to take where restaurant food is concerned. The psychology involved is that of a planned strategy and a freedom of personal choice for yourself. By allowing yourself this freedom, you may make some mistakes, but it may be better than feeling guilty and resentful of your diabetes and then making a habit of gorging to make up for it. In the final analysis, you must decide on the psychology and discipline that is right for you. Flexibility and good management skills are vitally important and will make for a happier and healthier diabetic.

5

Holiday Food

I promise to refrain from presenting a major dissertation on the subject of holiday food and diabetes. I am not trying to lecture or cajole you into compliance with the diabetic diet regime. Rather, we are brainstorming together in order to find the best solutions for you and your family as you deal with the diabetic diet and the daily ups and downs of living with diabetes.

One should try to focus on the positive aspects of the diabetic meal plan and to work with it in the most positive manner rather than to fight against it. I think you will find this strategy useful when holiday time rolls around and everyone is rather focused on eating all the wonderful foods that go so well with the festive season. It seems as though there is more of everything during the holidays — more candies, more desserts, more rich breads — thus making it difficult for the diabetic to regulate his or her diet. It is especially tempting, of course, when the aromas of homemade candies, pies, cakes, breads, turkey, ham, or roast beef begin drifting in from the kitchen, and the desire to eat in large quantities is triggered by the social gathering and the family talk. If you are the one who is cooking or helping with the cooking, it can be difficult to deal with the stress of preparing, handling, and sampling all that delicious food.

I view the holidays as a wonderful occasion to sample a great many tastes and aromas. Even though I enjoy this time of year immensely, I maintain my schedule as close to normal as I can, and I check my blood sugar for rises in my blood glucose due to my overeating of foods that I simply love, such as giblet dressing and cranberry salad loaded with pecans, fresh cranberries, navel orange pieces, and cherry Jell-O. Then there is the wonderful gravy for the dressing and the holiday roast. Oh, yes, do not forget the turkey or ham that seems to go so well with all these accouterments. Simply marvelous, right?

You can eat a little of all these wonderful items if you will simply remember one important factor, one we have talked about before. It is so simple, yet so difficult. We are talking about *quantity*. And we will talk about quantity again in other chapters of this book. Quantity seems to be the one thing that causes a problem for us diabetics. It is a double-edged sword that affects us by causing either too high a level of blood sugar (i.e., from eating too much) or too low a level of blood sugar (i.e., from eating too little). Again, this is a balancing act that is learned through experience and familiarity with the disease diabetes mellitus.

If you eat a large portion of the sweet cranberry salad, you are going to throw off your balance to the high side of the blood sugar scale. If you then follow your meal with a slice of pumpkin pie or pecan pie, your blood sugar just goes higher. What can you do? Yes, I know this is difficult, because remember, I go through these very same ups and downs every holiday season myself. But, you will find it best to eat only a bite or two of the sweet items, and more of the items that are not calorie intensive, such as tossed salad, sliced raw vegetables, pickles, and coleslaw. In this way, you can sample the wonderful-tasting, fattening items that everyone else is enjoying, but fill up on the items that will cause no significant rise in your blood sugar.

Remember that this is just one strategy that I use in dealing with holiday food. Perhaps you would prefer not to eat the foods that will cause your blood sugar to rise dramatically, and this is a fine method also. However, most people like to enjoy a few items during the holidays that make these days so special. I think you can enjoy these items as much as the nondiabetic folks out there and keep yourself in good diabetic control by careful planning for this time of year. We have developed a strategy for the party, for the restaurant, and now for the holiday season. You can see that these techniques are similar and merely require engagement in their specific application to be effective.

Overall good management of the situation is also required during these times. When a family gets together, whether it is a large family gathering or a small family gathering, the timing of the food is more critical for the diabetic than it is for the others. If, for instance, the main meal is not to be ready until three or four in the afternoon, a situation that seems to happen at my house, then the diabetic should have a snack during the normal lunchtime to prevent the low blood sugar reaction that may occur if the diabetic skips a meal or waits too long to eat. The holidays require a fine balancing act when it comes to timing the administration of the insulin dose, checking blood sugar, and timing meals.

It is important to remember that the diabetic must eat at regular intervals. What if the family wants to eat just one big meal for that day? Well, this is not possible for the diabetic. The diabetic must have something to eat for breakfast, lunch, and dinner, no matter what type of holiday is under way. Perhaps a smaller breakfast and lunch will do in order to save some calories for the big meal of the day; however, it is important to watch for insulin reactions. Orange juice should always be kept on hand for the diabetic who may suffer a low blood sugar reaction or insulin reaction. Orange juice acts quickly to reduce the effects of the insulin reaction. Again, monitoring your blood glucose and some common sense are the keys here.

Remember that foods prepared during the holiday season are usually made with rich ingredients. Generally, caution is thrown to the wind when it comes to using salt, real butter, heavy cream, and other fattening ingredients. Your particular strategy in dealing with the holiday season is important in living with your diabetes. Again, be a little flexible with yourself, use good common sense and logic in planning your strategy, and balance your diet wisely, and you will enjoy the season as much or more than the others.

Travel Food

*I*n this chapter we will look closely at some of the important issues involved in planning to travel with diabetes. These considerations should be kept in mind when traveling around the neighborhood, around town, or around the world.

Let us take a look at the following scenario: You and your husband plan a family picnic at the lake, which includes a two-hour drive to your favorite camping area. You pack up enough sandwiches, cold drinks, potato chips, sliced raw vegetables and pickles, salad, and fruit for a nice day. You remember to take along some extra insulin and syringes because it will be late in the evening when you return, and you will need your evening insulin dose. After getting the picnic and camping gear ready, you finally get the kids and all the gear packed away in the van for the drive. Because you had an adequate breakfast, including a high-fiber cereal, milk, orange juice, and some wheat toast with low-fat cream cheese, you feel quite confident that this should last you until you have lunch when you arrive at the lake. The various trips out to the van packing away the gear and a little additional stress when your husband could not find his fly-fishing rod and reel, mixed in with getting the sandwiches ready, all went unnoticed as the busy morning sped by. Indeed, this actually required more energy than you anticipated; however, the effort was well worth it and as you get into the passenger seat, with the kids safely in the back, the well-needed mini vacation is under way.

About thirty minutes out of town, your husband becomes nauseous and complains of a tremendous headache. He asks you to drive so he can gather his energy up for the rest of the trip. After you have been driving for almost an hour with the lake about thirty minutes away, all of a sudden you realize you are in a sweat. You feel a flush of panic, you have a headache, and you are slightly confused. Disoriented, but acutely aware that something is wrong, you pull the van over to the side of the road and get the container of orange juice you packed for the unexpected insulin reaction that has now begun to come on strong. As you drink the orange juice, the immediate effect of the sugar intake causes the insulin reaction to subside and the journey can resume.

Well, what is the lesson here? It is important to remember to take the orange juice or candy necessary for that unforeseen insulin reaction along with you on any trip. In the above example, the woman with insulin-dependent diabetes might have made the journey without an insulin reaction if she had not had to take over the driving. Driving is an activity that requires a great deal of attention, and as the energy consumption is increased during this activity, the demand for glucose (sugar) is also increased. If for some reason there had been no orange juice or other source of sugar available in the van, then the diabetic would have had to look for a convenience store or other area where a sugar soda could be obtained. If the family had been in an area where there were no stores, then without a source of glucose in the car, the diabetic would have been in trouble. The energy expended in packing up the van and getting everyone ready for the trip and then the additional burden of the driving all added up to cause the diabetic to fall into a hypoglycemic episode or what we call an insulin reaction. Furthermore, it is important for the diabetic to understand that if an accident should occur while he or she is experiencing an insulin reaction, the responsibility for this accident could fall squarely on the shoulders of the diabetic. It is up to the diabetic to maintain safety while operating a motor vehicle, and this responsibility includes proper control of the disease.

When going on a car trip, whether it is just a short trip or a major cross-country trip, be sure you carry enough sugar-containing products that will get you out of the dreaded insulin reaction. You could carry hard candies or other forms of candy, restaurant-style packets of sugar, orange juice or other high-sugar fruit juice that comes in the little drink boxes with straws attached to the sides, or cans of sugar soft drinks for the trip. I especially like to carry along with me the small drink boxes of real orange juice. I find that for me orange juice is the fastest-acting remedy for an insulin reaction, and it is very convenient to use. You may prefer to try something different; however, I would recommend you at least try orange juice, and always keep whatever product you choose on hand, as it may save your life.

Here is another scenario: You are planning a trip from Denver, Colorado, to San Diego, California. Your flight has been scheduled far in advance, and you are doing some planning in order to make the plane trip as smooth and enjoyable as possible. Depending on the time of departure from Denver, it will be important for you to know what kind of meal or snacks will be available to you on the airplane. Is this the type of fare-savings flight that will offer you only a bag of peanuts and a cold drink of some sort? If they will provide a snack, is it going to be a sandwich and fruit? If they are going to serve a hot meal, then what and when will it be? Once you know the meal schedule for your flight, you can prepare accordingly. If the flight will provide only peanuts, and your mealtime is during this flight, carry on a lunch bag for yourself with a sandwich and a piece of fruit. Would the airline make a special snack for a diabetic passenger if you requested them to do so? Many airlines are cognizant of the dietary requirements that some passengers have and will accommodate you, although some may not be able to do this. You should know in advance and plan to take care of yourself if the airline is not equipped to do so. Thankfully, the airlines do offer orange juice on their flights, and even the commuter flights will offer a quick beverage before touchdown.

Traveling through time zones may also present a management problem for you if you are under strict dietary control and timing. In the above example, if you are leaving Denver at 10:00 A.M., it is only 9:00 A.M. in San Diego. If the flight requires three hours for arrival, in Denver it is 1:00 P.M., while at the gate in San Diego, it is only 12:00 P.M. If you ate lunch on the plane, and it is now 12:00 P.M. — lunchtime in San Diego — when should you eat again? This is not a monumental problem when there is only a one-hour time differential, but what if you are flying around the world, and the timing is six hours different from your schedule? This does, indeed, require some planning and careful management of your diabetes and your food intake and timing. Doctors with experience in travel medicine advise the insulin-dependent diabetic to reduce his or her insulin intake when traveling to the east, in order to accommodate the shortened day. When traveling to the west, especially when traveling through three or four time zones, and the day is lengthened, an additional amount of insulin should be taken.

This tailoring of the insulin dose must be evaluated by your doctor. Most doctors agree that when traveling to the east, the insulin should be adjusted downward by two-thirds of the standard dose. When traveling to the west, taking an additional dose of one-third, after eighteen to twenty hours, may be helpful. Again, because adjustment of insulin dosage is an individual issue, consultation with your doctor is very important, and careful blood sugar monitoring should always be carried out. As a diabetic, it is very important for you to know the type of food that will be served during your flight, no matter how long it is. If your blood sugar should fall and you begin to feel the symptoms of an impending insulin reaction, rest assured that the flight attendant will be able to bring you orange juice or a sugar soft drink to bring you out of this situation. If you are traveling on a small commuter-type aircraft that may not have a beverage cart, you should bring your own juice.

I have done a lot of traveling and have been fortunate never to have suffered an insulin reaction during a flight, but many times I have had to inject myself with insulin on the plane. Planning is the key element again. I always monitor my blood glucose before any trip and eat an adequate meal before I leave for the airport. This is really not a difficult planning procedure and involves good common sense.

If you plan to take an extended trip to a foreign country, I strongly advise you to consult with your doctor and be well aware of the foods that will be available and the health conditions before you make the trip plans. As a diabetic in a foreign country, you should carry extra insulin and syringes or oral antidiabetic medication, along with pre-scriptions for each item. Then, should any unforeseen problem arise, you will be prepared. Remember, amoebic dysentery in a foreign country can represent a life-threatening situation for anyone. When diabetes is added in, the situation can become complicated very quickly. Most frequently, visitors to a foreign country will suffer travelers' diarrhea, which can make one extremely ill. The most important consideration here is to be informed about the foods and beverages that are likely to be contaminated and should be avoided. A saying that is very important to remember as a traveler in a foreign country is, "If you cannot cook it, boil it, or peel it, then forget it." In other words, foods must be well prepared, well cooked, and served steaming hot.

Generally, non-insulin-dependent diabetics will not encounter the degree of management problems that the insulin-dependent diabetic will encounter. Problems encountered by the traveling non-insulin-dependent diabetic may include eating too much. Another consideration for the non-insulin-dependent diabetic is getting less exercise than he or she would get at home. Good management of your own particular case of diabetes and careful note of any major change in symptoms is crucial. Consultation with your doctor is the best advice here. A visit to your doctor should be part of the trip planning and should include a thorough physical exam, a blood test, and whatever other tests your doctor deems necessary. Your plans for a trip abroad should be discussed with your doctor and careful note of any special advice should be taken.

In summing up, I think one point stands out above the rest. You should always carry a supply of sugar-containing products with you whether you are just driving to the store or driving across the state. Never let yourself get into a situation where you do not have some candy, sugar, or orange juice at your immediate disposal. Low blood sugar can be life-threatening and is therefore a major concern. As long as you are adequately prepared for this situation on any trip you plan to take, you will have covered a major base. Planning, strategy, and common sense, along with good blood sugar control and sensible eating, have been our watchwords for the chapters on party food and drink, restaurant food, holiday food, and now travel food. As you practice these management techniques over the long term, they will become part of your life.

7

How About a Late-Night Snack?

When I was a child I loved to read the Sunday comics. I always got a big charge out of reading "Blondie." I loved it when Dagwood went to the refrigerator and made a huge Dagwood sandwich late at night. I can still picture this sandwich, with multiple layers of bologna, salami, chicken legs, roast beef, cheese, hard-boiled eggs, and even fish, as well as anything else he could find in the refrigerator, between two pieces of bread, replete with an olive toothpicked on top. As I got older, I would joke to myself that Dagwood might be an uncontrolled diabetic with a voracious appetite and just had to satisfy a late-night craving for a snack. Indeed, over the years I have found myself going to the refrigerator late at night and piecing together a sandwich that would make Dagwood proud.

In most meal-planning programs for the insulin-dependent diabetic, the dietitian will factor in a snack before bedtime. The reason for this is to provide some additional calories for the body to rely on throughout the night and early hours of the next morning. When asleep, many diabetics will suffer a drop in blood sugar with a resulting insulin reaction that disturbs sleep, and if one is a heavy sleeper, this can represent a dangerous situation. The late-night snack provides some long-lasting protein, usually in the form of milk, cheese, and crackers, that will sustain the diabetic through the night.

If you are insulin-dependent and take multiple injections to control your blood sugar, then your doctor and dietitian may suggest that a snack before bedtime be included in your meal plan. Of course, this is another one of those areas where the individual's needs dictate the regimen, based upon the insulin intake, exercise, and caloric requirements. It is therefore impossible for me to suggest how much of a snack you may or may not require. If you are non-insulin-dependent and rely on strict dietary control in order to manage your diabetes, then a snack late at night may do more harm than good, in the form of weight gain, especially if your blood sugar does not fluctuate dramatically.

The diabetic can adjust his or her late-night snack based on the amount of food intake for the evening meal and a late-evening blood sugar reading. A good rule of thumb is to have at least a four- to six-ounce glass of milk to sustain you throughout the night. Milk is a protein and will metabolize slowly. If you were to eat a high-glucose load — for instance, a piece of candy or pie — this inrush of sugar would cause your blood sugar to rise dramatically. It is preferable to eat some form of protein, as in the milk, cheese, and crackers idea, that will break down slowly and maintain a more even blood sugar. Your dietitian may advise a small piece of fruit, such as half an apple or half an orange, to supplement your snack. Remember, your snack can be adjusted, and you can control how much you should eat based on your blood sugars and your activity level. If you are running consistently high morning blood sugars, then your intake at snack time may be too much. Again, this will have to be experimented with, and your dietitian can give some helpful hints for the best way to deal with a late-night snack.

I have been known to go wild with my late-night snack. Give me a brick of cheese, some wheat crackers, and a sharp knife, and my snack will turn into a high-calorie meal. Hey, this is a snack, remember, Joe? Yes, I did have a high blood sugar reading the next morning, and there was no wondering why, either. Try not to get carried away with the snack idea, like I sometimes do.

I have found that some low-fat cream cheese on wheat crackers makes an excellent snack. I try to dole out about five crackers and place a small amount of cream cheese on each. Then I put the cream cheese and the rest of the crackers away so that I will not be tempted to pig out. Another snack idea I like is sliced chicken or turkey on my crackers. Add a half glass of milk and it is wonderful.

There are many different combinations you can try. One of my favorites in years past was a marinated artichoke on Triscuit crackers. A slice of Danish ham with some cream cheese on a half piece of wheat bread is also very good. The key here is not to eat too much. The diabetic snack is something I have always secretly looked forward to having before I retire at night. It is a wonderful way to end the day. Obviously, Dagwood had the right idea.

8

Sweeteners

Glucose, dextrose, fructose, levulose, lactose, maltose, and sucrose . . . and then we have granulated sugar, confectioners' sugar, powdered sugar, turbinado sugar, brown sugar, corn sugar, corn syrup, honey, invert sugar, maple syrup, maple sugar, molasses, sorghum, and dextrin.

And have you ever heard of Sucanat? How about mannitol, sorbitol, and xylitol, the sugar alcohols? There are also the noncaloric, nonnutritive sweeteners: aspartame (NutraSweet, Equal, Spoonful), acesulfame-K (Sweet One), saccharin, and calcium saccharin (Sweet'n Low).

There do indeed seem to be a large number of sugars out there to confuse us diabetics. Let's look at them closely.

The sugars in the first group of terms above are the chemical names for the caloric, nutritive sweeteners. The second group includes the common names for the sugars we are all familiar with and use daily. The sugar alcohols, the third group, are sugars that you may not be familiar with, and the fourth group, the artificial sweeteners, are the noncaloric, nonnutritive sweeteners that diabetics and those wishing to reduce caloric intake find so helpful.

Nutritive Sweeteners with Chemical Names

First, let us begin with the sugars with chemical names ending in *ose*, the caloric, nutritive sweeteners. If you add these to your diet, you should consult with your dietitian and carefully account for the calories they will add.

Glucose is the basic simple sugar found in the blood. You have read in this book many times the statement "Be sure to check your blood sugar regularly." Normal blood glucose is measured at 70 to 110 milligrams per deciliter (mg/dl). In diabetes mellitus, free glucose is found in levels much higher than normal in blood and urine. Glucose is either absorbed from digested food or manufactured from all the various sugars as well as from carbohydrates, fats, and protein. Another name for glucose is dextrose.

Fructose is fruit sugar. It is a very sweet sugar found in fruit, honey, and juices. It is not obtained from fruit, but is produced by chemically splitting sucrose into its simple sugars, glucose and fructose, and then isolating and purifying the fructose. Liquid fructose, or high-fructose corn syrup, is made by treating corn syrup with enzymes to convert some of its starch to fructose. Fructose has become available as a tabletop sweetener and is used by some diabetics. It is as sweet or sweeter than sucrose and has no nutritive value. Commercially, fructose is found in granular and liquid forms, but if you decide to use it, be aware of the different concentrations that are available. What is called "pure" fructose is 90 percent fructose. Fifty-five percent fructose is high-fructose corn syrup, which contains a large percentage of glucose. In diabetic individuals with well-controlled diabetes, it will cause less of a blood sugar rise than glucose or sucrose. This is so because after leaving the digestive tract and entering the liver, fructose is either used immediately or stored as glycogen (stored glucose). Poorly controlled diabetics experience a significant rise in blood sugar after ingesting fructose, due to the liver's quick conversion of fructose into free glucose. Research into the role of fructose and its use by the diabetic, and its implication for weight gain and effect on triglyceride levels, continues. Levulose is just another name for fructose.

Lactose is milk sugar. Occurring naturally, lactose is a disaccharide — two sugars linked together — present in mammalian milk and obtained from milk and milk products, such as cheese, ice cream, and yogurt. Lactose intolerance is a medical condition wherein the body does not have the enzymes necessary to break down this sugar.

Maltose, or malt sugar, is a crystalline sugar formed by the breakdown of starch.

Sucrose is refined sugar that is used in cooking and added to foods at the table. Ordinary sucrose is a combination of two sugars, glucose and fructose, chemically bonded together in equal amounts to produce sucrose. In order to produce sucrose, glucose and fructose must be chemically extracted from sugarcane or sugar beets and refined through a series of steps.

Nutritive Sweeteners with Common Names

Granulated sugar, also called table sugar, is added at the table and in cooking. It is a sweet sugar, sucrose. Confectioners' sugar, sucrose, is a sweet powdery sugar used most often in cooking. It is also known as powdered sugar. Turbinado sugar is raw sugar that has been steam cleaned and contains some molasses. Brown sugar, sucrose, is a sweet, soft sugar whose crystals are covered by a film of refined hard syrup. Corn sugar is a sugar made from the breakdown of cornstarch; corn syrup is a syrup containing several different sugars obtained by the partial breakdown of cornstarch, maltose, and other glucose molecules.

Honey, man's first concentrated sweetener, is a very sweet, thick syrup made up mostly of fructose. Due to honey's popularity and trace quantities of nutrients, many diabetics believe that it can be easily substituted for sugar or other sweeteners. But because honey is highly concentrated glucose, it is not a good choice for the diabetic, and its intake should generally be avoided.

Invert sugar is a combination of sugars found in fruit. Through a process called inversion, sucrose is treated with acid in order to produce invert sugar. Maple syrup is a syrup made by concentrating the sap of a sugar maple. Maple sugar is a candy made from maple syrup.

Molasses is a thick, dark to light brown liquid sugar that is separated from raw sugar in its manufacturing. Sorghum is a syrup from the sweet juice of the sorghum grain.

Dextrin is a sugar formed from the partial breakdown of starch. It is a mixture of glucose molecules formed during the enzymatic breakdown or acid hydrolysis of starch, pectin, or glycogen. Upon further hydrolysis, it is converted into glucose.

Sucanat is a granular, crystalline sugar produced from organically grown sugarcane. Its name is derived from "*sugarcane natural.*" Sucanat was developed about twenty years ago by a Swiss pediatrician who wanted a pure sugar product for his patients as an alternative to white sugar. Nothing is added to Sucanat; only the water is removed so that all the complex sugars and the molasses are retained. Pesticide and chemical free, Sucanat is pure sugar, so be cautious, as with other nutritive sweeteners, with your level of intake.

Sugar Alcohols

The sugar alcohols, mannitol, sorbitol, and xylitol, are sugars commonly used in manufacturing, and are sometimes referred to as polyols. These caloric sweeteners contain an alcohol group (−OH), denoted by the use of a terminal *ol* in their names. These sweeteners provide gram for gram about the same amount of calories as other caloric sweeteners. The sugar alcohols have been shown to cause the blood sugar to rise more slowly after their ingestion than glucose or sucrose, and therefore less insulin response is elicited. All three of the sugar alcohols, when eaten in large quantities (twenty to fifty grams a day for adults, five to ten grams for children), may cause diarrhea. A single piece of dietetic candy may have three grams of sorbitol.

Mannitol is metabolized in the same way as other sugars, but absorbed more slowly. Sorbitol is a crystalline sugar formed by the breakdown of starch. Xylitol is a naturally occurring sugar alcohol made from xylose, which is bark sugar.

Noncaloric, Nonnutritive Sweeteners

Aspartame, trade named NutraSweet, is the generic name for one of the most popular artificial sweeteners today. It is one of the ingredients found in Equal (available in individual blue packets). Aspartame contains amino acids, phenylalanine, and aspartic acid. With an excellent sweet taste and no aftertaste, it has become the artificial sweetener of choice. Because even a small amount of aspartame is extremely sweet, it provides only a few calories. NutraSweet is now found in diet soft drinks, desserts, ice cream, candy, and many other items that rely on a very good-tasting noncaloric agent for sweetness. I use Equal often in coffee and iced tea and find it to be a very pleasant sweetening agent. If you are accustomed to the high sweetness of saccharin, Equal may not be sweet enough for you if you use only one packet. You may want to try an additional one-quarter to one-half packet for the level of sweetness you desire.

There is a trick to using aspartame in cooking. Because it is a protein and tends to break down easily, it will lose its sweetness when cooked for long periods. So it is best to add aspartame to a cooked item after it has cooled.

Many questions have been raised as to the safety of aspartame. Research indicates that it is a safe product even when consumed at abusive levels, unless one is sensitive to phenylalanine. Persons with phenylketonuria (PKU) should not use this product without the advice of their doctors. It is my opinion that even though research indicates the relative safety of this product, moderation is still a key watchword. The U.S. Food and Drug Administration (FDA) and most doctors feel that aspartame is safe when used moderately.

A new aspartame sweetener trade named Spoonful, made by the manufacturers of NutraSweet, is now available on grocers' shelves. This is a granulated sugar substitute approved by the FDA in February 1992. It is said that Spoonful, teaspoon for teaspoon, looks, tastes, and measures just like sugar. Spoonful is made from aspartame and maltodextrin, with only two calories per teaspoon, while sugar has about sixteen calories per teaspoon. The unique quality of Spoonful is that you can use it just as you would sugar, in desserts and sprinkled over cereal and fruit.

The newest artificial sweetener on the block is acesulfame-potassium, or acesulfame-K. As a tabletop sweetener, acesulfame-K is marketed under the trade name Sweet One. Acesulfame-K is very concentrated, tasting about two hundred times as sweet as sugar; each packet equals two teaspoons of sugar. Chemically, it is similar to saccharin but is clean tasting with no aftertaste. It may taste bitter, however, if used in high concentrations. Acesulfame-K can be used in baking and cooking, as it does not break down under heat. The FDA says that acesulfame-K is safe to use. Unfortunately, as with many of the artificial sweeteners, it will not give the same texture to baked goods that sugar does. Some cooks will use a small amount of sugar along with the artificial sweetener in order to have good texture and a nice finished product.

Saccharin is an artificial sweetener that contains no carbohydrate and is approximately 375 times sweeter than sucrose. The FDA has tried to ban the use of saccharin since 1977, due to well-publicized research on laboratory animals that were given tremendously high quantities of saccharin. It was reported that these animals, in some cases, developed bladder adenomas and associated cancerous lesions. This research was controversial due to the large quantities of saccharin these animals ingested. The American Diabetes Association and many experts have questioned the action of the FDA, considering the benefits received by millions of diabetics and others who use saccharin. Also, for many of us who were diagnosed with diabetes before the development of the new generation of artificial sweeteners such as aspartame, saccharin was the only sweetener to choose from, as cyclamates had been taken off the market in the early 1970s. Congress has repeatedly extended a law that prohibits banning saccharin. The American Diabetes Association feels that a ban on saccharin is unjustified and has recommended that food safety laws be amended to allow the government to further evaluate food additives, including saccharin, on the basis of their risks and benefits.

Sweet'n Low, a product of Kraft Foods (available in individual pink packets), is a combination nutritive and nonnutritive sweetener. It has four calories per packet, which come from dextrose, the nutritive sweetener. The nonnutritive component is calcium saccharin. I have used this particular product for years and find it to be very sweet. For some, it may produce a characteristic aftertaste, and use of less than an entire packet may be advisable.

During the late 1980s some research suggested that artificial sweeteners used in sodas, gum, and candies have an overall effect of increasing hunger. There were several studies conducted that shed very little light as to a clear-cut answer to this rather paradoxical situation. Dr. Barbara Rowles, an associate professor of psychiatry at Johns Hopkins University, found, after an exhaustive review of the literature and research on artificial sweeteners, that they have never been found to increase food intake. Research done by Rowles determined that nonsugar sweeteners increased neither hunger nor food intake, and by allowing consumption of palatable foods that would otherwise have to be avoided, they could be useful in dieting.

I am glad the research was done on that area of controversy concerning artificial sweeteners. I have been able to enjoy artificially sweetened soft drinks that would have been off limits to me if only sugar-sweetened soft drinks were available. I remember the time only too well when we had to round up a saccharin pill or two, usually carried in a small pillbox, for addition to iced tea. It was amazing how insoluble these tiny saccharin pills could be as you took your iced tea spoon and tried to smash them into pieces at the bottom of your glass. You can now find artificial sweeteners at any restaurant, and it certainly is convenient to simply tear open a small envelope containing a very soluble artificial sweetener, stir, and enjoy.

The Sweet Conclusion

It is up to you to carefully monitor your sugar intake. Read ingredients lists. A food with caloric sweeteners at the beginning of the list is sure to be high in sugar. If there are other sugars farther down the list, the combination all adds up to a lot of sugar. I have read cereal packages that list brown sugar, corn syrup, molasses, and fructose in the ingredients list, which means that this type of cereal will most likely cause extremely high blood sugar. In the final analysis, it is your choice which sweetener to use and how much. As with all aspects of diabetes, moderation and balance is the wise choice, and with sweets and sweeteners, this is doubly so.

9

Diabetics and Desserts

In the not so recent past desserts were a strictly forbidden topic for diabetics; even thinking about sweets was completely out of the question. This was especially hard for all of us who really love something sweet at the end of a meal.

But with today's sweeteners that taste almost like real sugar and with a new philosophy that the intake of carbohydrates can be liberalized, we diabetics now have a far greater range of choices. We also have ultrasmall blood glucose meters that are easily carried in pocket or purse, which enable us to monitor and control our blood sugars to a much finer degree than ever before.

Most people like to eat something sweet once in a while. Of course, some people absolutely crave sweets in all forms, while some people can do without them easily. If you are one of those who desire sweet desserts, but now have diabetes, I think the first step is to admit to the fact that you still do like them, and that life would seem rather boring if you were totally deprived. And furthermore, unless you are practicing the ascetic lifestyle of a monk, you will want to enjoy a dessert on occasion.

The rationale is this: If you allow yourself to enjoy a sweet dessert once in a while, then the tendency to develop frustration and bitterness toward your diabetes will diminish. But if you place yourself on a totally restrictive program excluding desserts entirely, you may find yourself resenting your diabetes, and if and when your willpower succumbs, you may pig out on sweets or other foods that are not good for you. I find that eating a small amount of sweet desserts occasionally does no harm, and does not significantly alter the course of my diabetic meal plan. Today's modified diet for the diabetic and new thinking in terms of more liberalized carbohydrate intake allow us to take this moderate approach to sweets.

When I get together with friends for dinner and everyone orders a dessert, I find it very easy to refuse a dessert if I so choose. However, if I should choose to have a dessert, I will enjoy it as much as the others, but I will allow myself to have only a few bites, never the entire dessert. This way, I am able to enjoy the sweet taste at the end of the meal, without the high blood sugar that comes with eating too much.

Learning to live moderately presents a complex problem for an inexperienced Type II diabetic who craves sugary desserts but needs to maintain the diabetic diet and meal plan. Many doctors throw up their hands in defeat in cases of newly diagnosed Type II non-insulin-dependent elderly diabetic patients who are faced with the learning curve that all beginning diabetics must adapt to. On the one hand, if the Type II diabetic refrains from eating sweets and assiduously maintains a healthful low-fat diet, it may be possible for him or her to improve to the point of not even needing oral antidiabetic medication. On the other hand, if this person does not maintain a carefully managed diabetic diet and splurges with sweet desserts and candies all the time, then he or she may face becoming rediagnosed with Type I insulin-dependent diabetes, or, in other words, having to take daily insulin injections.

I have a dear friend who is sixty-five years old and was diagnosed with non-insulin-dependent diabetes mellitus two years ago. She finds it terribly difficult to live without desserts after years of really enjoying pecan pie, chocolate cake, homemade peanut brittle, homemade ice cream, cheesecake, cherry cobbler, and the like. This is the kind of deprivation that brings on what she and I call a "DD day," a "that damned disease day" that gives you the blues.

This is why I feel you should not be too hard on yourself; total denial of all desserts may lead to emotional and psychological trouble. Defining the limits of dessert intake for yourself will be by trial and error, but try to maintain the balance that seems to be so crucial in diabetes management.

10

A Word About Fiber, Fiber, Fiber

Diabetes is a most complex disease. Where would the disease be today if over fifty years ago diabetics were afforded the new highly purified and refined human insulins and new medications that are now available, along with the ability to self-monitor one's blood sugars through home blood glucose monitors? Speculating further along this line, where will the health of the diabetic population be in the next fifty years if a diet high in fiber is entered into today?

There are several things that I now lament not having done for myself in years past as a diabetic. One of these items is not starting sooner on a meticulous program of tight blood sugar control. I was trained to care for my diabetes in a program of rather loose control that did not stress normalizing the blood glucose. Of course, in those days, we did not have home blood glucose monitors, which have revolutionized the control level of diabetes. I also lament not entering into a high-fiber diet fifteen years ago. Although I am a big advocate of fiber today, and I am in very good health for a diabetic in his third decade with this disease, I wonder if entering into a high-fiber diet earlier would have lessened the severity or retarded the onset of diabetic retinopathy, the disease that caused me to become totally blind.

You may be thinking, "But how can you make the correlation between high dietary-fiber intake and the onset of a long-term complication of insulin-dependent diabetes?" Indeed, due to the extremely complex nature of microvascular disease within long-term diabetes, microangiopathy, it is merely speculation on my part that a high-fiber diet may increase the possibility of reducing the severity of this disease state by helping to reduce the accumulation of fat and cholesterol within the arteries.

One of the most difficult problems we face as diabetics is the destruction of our blood vessels through the degradation of micro- and macrovascular disease. This is an insidious and long-term process, aided and abetted by the diabetes itself, and a myriad of other disease processes that accompany and are a part of diabetes.

If one were able to prevent clogged arteries (atherosclerosis), hardening of the arteries (arteriosclerosis), and the formation of plaques of cholesterol and fatty deposits (hypercholesterolemia, hypertriglyceridemia, and hyperlipidemia), what would be the overall effect on the target organs that diabetes so ravages, such as the eyes and kidneys? In becoming serious about the diabetic diet, these questions must be considered and long thought given to the best positive attitude when the decision is made to accept the challenge of living with diabetes and utilizing the diet as an integral part of the therapy regime designed to prolong your life.

The incidence of diabetes seems to be quite high all over the world except in some areas, such as rural Africa, where the incidence is low. Why is this? In parts of the world where there is a large dietary intake of unrefined foods, fruits, and vegetables, and an almost total lack of fat, sugar, and meat, there is very little, if any, diabetes. As scientists began studying eating behavior, it was seen again and again that in areas of high dietary-fiber intake, the incidence of diabetes was low. In areas where there was little dietary-fiber intake, the incidence of diabetes was high.

It has become alarmingly evident that Americans do not include enough fiber in their diets. A great deal of research has been undertaken to show the relationship between high dietary-fiber intake and the reduced risk of coronary heart disease, atherosclerosis, arteriosclerosis, stroke, digestive diseases, and diabetes. Studies show that the intake of dietary fiber really does reduce the risk and severity of these diseases.

What is fiber? The fiber that we are talking about is plant fiber. In the natural state, all the plants we use for food have fiber that is part of the plant tissue. Dietary fiber is the nondigestible carbohydrates, including pectin, cellulose, endocellulose, and lignin, which make up the cell walls of plants. In its natural state, the purpose of plant fiber tissue is to help the plant grow, retain vital nutrients, and heal and protect itself when damaged.

Fiber is found most abundantly in raw, leafy, and tough-skinned vegetables; fruits; edible seeds; nuts; and the outer layer of grains. As the human digestive system does not have the essential bacteria needed to break down fiber, it remains more or less unchanged and is passed out of the body through the gastrointestinal system. Dietary fiber has a great capacity to absorb water, which gives bulk to the system, softens the stool, and allows easy elimination through the system.

During the last three decades, the food processing industry has rushed to remove fiber from food to make it more convenient to eat. We have fallen victim to fast foods, convenience, the super technology of refining, and precooking. The removal of fiber from our most often consumed foods, such as the husks from grains and rice, and the removal of fiber from fruits and vegetables through commercial processing has caused some changes in the manner in which the body derives nourishment.

You can prove this fact for yourself. First, check your blood sugar to establish a baseline for this simple test. Then drink a four-ounce glass of apple juice and thirty minutes later check your blood sugar again. The following day, check your blood sugar to establish a baseline as you did the preceding day. Then, eat a large apple, wait thirty minutes, and test your blood sugar again. You will find that the apple, with the natural fruit fiber and juice, will not cause your blood sugar to rise as dramatically as did the apple juice alone. This is one of fiber's most important roles for the diabetic. In this case, the fiber in the apple actually slowed down the absorption of carbohydrates, thus preventing a dramatic rise in the blood sugar. Generally, blood sugar values are lower after ingesting a meal high in dietary fiber. These important factors, along with the ability of fiber, specifically soluble fiber, to directly or indirectly reduce blood fat — triglycerides — which is partly responsible for heart disease and other vascular complications, are part of the reasons why fiber is so important for the diabetic.

Fiber creates a feeling of fullness, thus helping to prevent overeating. This is important for the non-insulin-dependent diabetic, as this extra bulk helps to cut back on calories without making one feel hungry and starved. Because fiber slows down the absorption of sugar through the gut, the blood sugar is evened out, as in the example above comparing apple juice with an apple. For the non-insulin-dependent diabetic, this slowing down of the transfer of sugar means that a high-insulin response is avoided. By avoiding the high-insulin response, feelings of hunger several hours after eating are also avoided.

For the insulin-dependent diabetic, fiber helps to even out the blood sugar highs and lows that are a part of this type of diabetes by slowing the absorption of carbohydrates in the gut. For many insulin-dependent diabetics, addition of dietary fiber provides the benefit of reducing insulin requirements. I have found this to be true for myself. With the addition of twenty grams of soluble fiber and five grams of insoluble fiber per day to my diet, I have been able to reduce my insulin intake by six units per day. Also — and this is very important — I have been able to maintain more normalized blood sugar values than ever before.

There are two types of fiber, soluble and insoluble. Simply stated, soluble fiber is fiber that goes completely into solution, or completely dissolves, when added to water. Water-soluble fiber can be found in oat bran and legumes and other vegetables, such as black-eyed peas, lima beans, kidney beans, navy beans, pinto beans, carrots, green peas, and corn. Broccoli, sweet potatoes, and zucchini have some soluble fiber, as do pears, bananas, oranges, apples, and prunes. Insoluble fiber is fiber that does not go into solution, or does not completely dissolve, when added to water. Insoluble fiber is found in wheat bran, whole wheat, most other whole grains, and most fruits and vegetables. Insoluble fiber is important for your digestive system and may help to prevent colon cancer, whereas water-soluble fiber is good for both digestion and possibly lowering blood cholesterol.

To better understand solubility, picture an eight-ounce glass of water to which you have added a tablespoon of salt. When stirred, the salt dissolves and goes completely into solution; i.e., salt is soluble in water. Now, picture an eight-ounce glass of water to which you have added a tablespoon of sand. When stirred, the sand is dispersed, but it will not go into solution no matter how hard you stir; therefore, sand is insoluble in water. Insoluble fiber can be thought of in much the same way, because when stirred, it is suspended in water, but when the stirring action stops, it will fall to the bottom of the glass and remain undissolved.

Although fiber is not digested by the human body, the benefits of adding both soluble and insoluble fiber to your diet are well established. Because fiber is such an important topic today, I will explain the mode of action of soluble fiber in terms of physiology and the benefits to your health.

All fiber, whether soluble or not, when taken in by mouth remains undigested material. When you eat a meal with fat in it, the food travels down the esophagus and into the stomach. Various enzymes do their part in the stomach to further break down the ingested food, compress and mix the food with fluid, and pass it along to the small intestine. In the small intestine, the food must be absorbed or it will do the body no good. A message is sent to the gallbladder, which is the storage bladder for bile. The liver makes bile, but it is stored in the gallbladder. The fat molecules are too large to be absorbed within the small intestine, so a message is sent to the gallbladder because help is needed to break the fat molecules into smaller and smaller pieces for eventual absorption. The gallbladder then squeezes bile out into the intestine. The bile then breaks these large fat molecules down and now you have absorption of fat by the gut. Additionally, with the absorption of fat is the reabsorption of bile.

When soluble fiber is added to the diet, it forms a gel in the gut. It acts like a protective film, and as the bile breaks the large fat molecules down, the soluble fiber gel coats the large fat molecules. In this way, the fiber gel prevents the fat and bile from being absorbed through the gut. The soluble fiber gel–fat molecule–bile complex is then passed out with a bowel movement. The prevention of fat absorption by soluble fiber is why the addition of this type of fiber is so important for the diabetic. By preventing reabsorption of bile, the enterohepatic circulation (*entero* meaning "gut," *hepatic* meaning "liver") is broken, thus preventing bile from returning to the liver to make more cholesterol. A diet high in soluble fiber breaks a cycle that is an important step in cholesterol synthesis.

Oat bran is an integral part of our discussion on fiber. In studies where reductions in cholesterol were dramatic, up to 19 percent, subjects ate a bowl of oatmeal and five oat bran muffins daily. This diet has proved to be rather difficult to remain on for very long. Incorporation of oat bran, leafy vegetables, and fruit into your diabetic diet should help to decrease your total blood cholesterol.

When shopping for products with oat bran, be sure to study carefully the level and type of oat bran contained in the product you are considering for purchase. Oats should be the first ingredient. Oats and other grains contain a small amount of fat in the natural state, but it is primarily unsaturated fat. You will want to avoid oat bran products that contain saturated fats or hydrogenated oils, as they may cancel out the benefits derived from the oat bran. Remember, saturated fats and hydrogenated oils will raise blood cholesterol.

In general, plain oatmeal and plain oat bran cereals are better sources of soluble fiber than are processed foods. Steel-cut, rolled, quick-cooking, and instant oats have the same amount of soluble fiber per gram, and the finer the cut the quicker the cereal cooks.

Studies have shown that diets high in soluble fiber reduce the risk of cardiovascular disease, the nation's number one killer. With the addition of insoluble fiber, the benefits of a clean colon mean more health benefits for the diabetic.

I derive fiber from fresh fruits and vegetables and take supplementary fiber, both soluble and insoluble. You should consult with your doctor and dietitian about entering into a high-fiber diet. I have found Metamucil, Citrucel, and Konsil D to be very useful in supplementing my fiber intake. I also use a high-nutrition, low-protein milk shake that has a proprietary formulation of soluble fiber once or twice a day. With the new thinking about fiber and the health benefits that can be derived, it is my opinion that you should investigate this area of nutrition for yourself, discuss this with your doctor, and rethink your diet in terms of including a higher fiber content.

Also a high-fiber diet should include drinking plenty of water and fluids.

For more information about fiber in your diet, consult *The Agriculture Handbook, Composition of Foods, Raw, Processed and Prepared*; chapter 1 of Betty Wedman's *American Diabetes Association Holiday Cookbook*; James Anderson's excellent book *Diabetes: A New Guide to Healthy*

Living; and *The High Fiber Cookbook for Diabetics* by Mabel Cavaiani. You will find full information about these sources in the Selected Reading List on pages 388–94.

The following list includes sources of oat bran fiber, fiber supplements, and nutrition formulations that include fiber. This list is not intended to be all-inclusive but is intended to give you some idea about sources of fiber other than fruits and vegetables.

Oat Bran Fiber Sources

Cereals

Old Fashioned Quaker Oats
Manufacturer: Quaker
Fiber per serving: 2.7 grams
Contents: oats; no artificial ingredients or additives; can be
    ground up in blender for addition to soups and sauces, and
    for making oat flour that can be used to make breads and
    muffins

Quaker Instant Oatmeal
Manufacturer: Quaker
Fiber per serving: 2 grams
Contents: oats and some additives; flavored varieties contain
    some fat and sugar and are high in sodium

Instant Oatmeal
Manufacturer: Arrowhead Mills
Fiber per serving: 4 grams
Contents: oats

Thirty-Second Oatmeal
Manufacturer: Napo

Fiber per serving: 2.5 grams
Contents: oats, wheat flour, and rye flour; fortified with iron

Cheerios
Manufacturer: General Mills
Fiber per serving: 2 grams
Contents: whole grain oat flour; fortified with vitamins and minerals

Oat Bran O's
Manufacturer: Health Valley
Fiber per serving: 2.8 grams
Contents: fruit juices, oats, and oat bran, along with other grains

Cracklin' Oat Bran
Manufacturer: Kellogg
Fiber per serving: 5 grams
Contents: oat bran, wheat bran, brown sugar, corn syrup, and dextrose, along with coconut and coconut oil; high in saturated fat

Breads

Oatmeal Bread (1½-pound loaf)
Manufacturer: Pepperidge Farms
Fiber per 1-slice serving: 1.5 grams
Contents: white flour, wheat flour, and some oatmeal

Bran'nola Country Oat Bread
Manufacturer: Arnold
Fiber per 1-slice serving: 3 grams

Contents: white flour, wheat flour, and oats; oat fiber, pea fiber, corn fiber, and wheat bran

Five Star Fiber Harvest Wheat Bread
Manufacturer: Pepperidge Farms
Fiber per 1-slice serving: 2.5 grams
Contents: white flour, wheat flour, oats, and other grains

Crackers

Seven Grain Vegetable Stone Wheat Crackers
Manufacturer: Health Valley
Fiber per 1-ounce serving: 2.75 grams
Contents: whole wheat flour, amaranth, barley malt, and oats; high in polyunsaturated fats, safflower oil

Oat Bran Graham Crackers
Manufacturer: Health Valley
Fiber per 1-ounce serving: 3 grams
Contents: whole wheat flour, oat bran, soy oil, and fruit juice

Fiber Supplements

Citrucel, 100% Soluble Fiber
Manufacturer: Merrill Dow Pharmaceutical
Fiber per teaspoon: 2 grams methylcellulose per rounded teaspoon
Mix 1 to 2 teaspoons with 8 ounces of water
Contents: active ingredient: methylcellulose (soluble fiber component); inactive ingredients: citric acid, F, D, and C yellow number 6, orange flavors, potassium citrate, riboflavin,

sucrose, or NutraSweet in nonnutritive formulation; 60 calories per rounded teaspoon

Metamucil, Orange Flavor, Sugar-Free
Manufacturer: Procter and Gamble
Fiber per teaspoon: 3.4 grams psyllium hydrophilic mucilloid
    per rounded teaspoon
Mix 1 to 2 teaspoons with 8 ounces of water
Contents: active ingredient: psyllium hydrophilic mucilloid (insoluble fiber component); inactive ingredients: aspartame, citric acid, F, D, and C yellow number 6, D and C yellow number 10, flavoring, and maltodextrin; 10 calories per rounded teaspoon

Konsil D
Manufacturer: Konsil Pharmaceutical
Fiber per teaspoon: 3.4 grams psyllium hydrophilic mucilloid
Mix 1 to 2 teaspoons with 8 ounces of water
Contents: active ingredient: psyllium hydrophilic mucilloid (insoluble fiber component); inactive ingredient: dextrose; 14 calories per 6.5-gram serving

Fiber-Containing Nutrition Drinks

The following two fiber-rich milk shake formulations are my personal favorites. I first began using Ultra Slim Fast, available on grocers' shelves, several years ago, enjoying the convenience of a high-fiber milk shake for breakfast. Ultra Slim Fast contains 4 grams of dietary fiber per serving. Although the addition of skim milk will add some calories, it fortifies the vitamin-rich shake and makes for an enjoyable breakfast. Note carefully the quantity of sugar found in Ultra Slim Fast.

The NANCI Lose It formulation, available only through special distributors, has 7.3 grams of fiber per serving, of which 90 percent is soluble and 10 percent is insoluble. This means that there is substantially more soluble fiber contained in this product than the insoluble dietary fiber found in Ultra Slim Fast. The Ultra Slim Fast product contains no soluble fiber, but relies on insoluble dietary fiber as its fiber agent. Dextrose and aspartame are the main sweetening ingredients in NANCI Lose It.

As both products contain a large quantity of fiber, I would suggest that unless you are accustomed to high fiber intake already, you work up to this level of daily fiber slowly, choosing one or the other of these milk shake formulations.

They also contain a high level of vitamins and, depending upon your own personal taste, will offer a nice change of pace for breakfast, or whichever meal you choose to substitute. Because these products are basically offered as high-fiber, high-nutrition weight loss programs, be sure to drink a lot of water along with your fiber drink and test your blood sugar often to ensure good glycemic control.

Ultra Slim Fast, Vanilla Flavor
Manufacturer: Slim Fast Foods
Fiber per 1-scoop serving (1.6 ounces): 4 grams dietary
   fiber
Mix 1 scoop with 8 ounces of skim milk
Contents: Protein (sources are one or more of nonfat dry
   milk, whey powder, soy protein isolate, whey protein
   concentrate, calcium caseinate), carbohydrates (sucrose,
   fructose, maltodextrin, dextrose), fiber (purified cellulose,
   corn bran, carrageenan, guar gum), lecithin, citric acid, d,
   methionine, aspartame, natural and artificial flavors and col-

ors, and the following vitamins and minerals: calcium phosphate, magnesium oxide, potassium chloride, ferric orthophosphate, ascorbic acid, vitamin E acetate, niacinamide, vitamin A palmitate, zinc oxide, manganese sulfate, calcium pantothenate, copper sulfate, vitamin D_3, pyridoxine hydrochloride, thiamine mononitrate, riboflavin, folic acid, biotin, potassium iodide, and vitamin B_{12}

NANCI

Manufacturer: NANCI Corporation

Fiber per serving: varying amounts for different age formulations; Lose It adult formulation, 7.3 grams dietary fiber

Mix 2 slightly rounded scoops with 8 ounces of water, fruit juice, or skim milk

Contents: soluble dietary fiber, nonfat dry milk (whey, nondairy creamer, corn syrup solids, partially hydrogenated canola oil, sodium caseinate, di-potassium phosphate, mono- and diglycerides, sodium silico aluminate, artificial flavor and color), powdered cellulose, sodium carboxymethyl-cellulose, artificial flavor, dextrose, calcium caseinate, tricalcium phosphate, canola oil, magnesium oxide, aspartame, ascorbic acid, alpha tocopheryl acetate, manganese sulfate, ferrous fumarate, zinc sulfate, niacin, vitamin A acetate, calcium pantothenate, pyridoxine hydrochloride, potassium chloride, copper oxide, riboflavin, thiamin mononitrate, vitamin D, folic acid, biotin, chromium chloride, potassium iodide, sodium molybdenate, sodium selenite, cyanocobalamin (vitamin B_{12})

Here is my favorite way to start the day in order to get a large amount of fiber into my diet:

Cranberry Acerola Super Shake

2 scoops vanilla NANCI Lose It
2 to 4 500 mg acerola chewable vitamin C tablets
8 ounces cranberry juice
4 to 6 ice cubes

Blend until thoroughly mixed, pour, and enjoy.

11

A Review of the Guidelines for Good Nutrition

L et us review briefly the nutritional guidelines and how good nutrition fits in with the addition of fiber to the diet. These guidelines have been designed by experts for the federal government and set forth to promote healthful eating and reduce the risk of food-related diseases within the general population. These guidelines are also part of the recommendations for principles of good nutrition by the American Diabetes Association (see chapter 2, "The Importance of the Diabetic Diet") and are appropriate for both adults and children.

1. The diet should be varied and include all food groups.

There are fifty known nutrients that the body needs to maintain a good state of health. No single food or food group will contain all the necessary nutrients. The more varied and balanced your diet becomes, the less likely you will be to develop a deficiency or excess of any nutrient. A varied diet also reduces the risk of exposure to contaminants within our food chain, which seems to be so prevalent today.

It is important to choose foods from the major food groups. The new chart put out by the federal government is a pyramid that gives recommended numbers of servings from five food groups. Bread, cereal, rice, and pasta form the largest group at the base of the pyramid; these complex carbohydrates are high in fiber and this group of foods should be consumed in highest quantity. The next level contains the vegetable and fruit groups. The milk, yogurt, and cheese group and the meat, poultry, fish, dried beans, eggs, and nuts group make up the third smaller level. The smallest level at the tip of the pyramid indicates that fats, oils, and sweets should be included in the diet in the least quantity.

2. In order to achieve proper weight, caloric intake and exercise should be adjusted to the individual.

Calories are the basic measurement of units of energy taken in and used up by the body. Fat is the result of eating food with more calories than the body can use; that is, unused calories are converted into fat. Fat is the main storage depot for energy. To give you an idea of the caloric requirement, in order to lose 1 pound of fat, you must cut 3,500 calories from your food intake. Exercise will also help in reducing fat through the utilization of these excess calories. For the diabetic, excess fat should be strictly avoided.

3. Limit fat and consumption of high-fat foods.

Fatty foods pose more than just a weight problem. It has now been well established that fat, especially saturated fat, and foods high in cholesterol are the primary contributors to heart disease and other vascular diseases. Because diabetes in and of itself accelerates these disease processes, the addition of high dietary fat makes a bad problem worse. The average American gets 40 to 50 percent of his or her total calories from fat. It is recommended that this be reduced to 30 percent of total calories.

4. Increase intake of complex carbohydrates and limit intake of simple carbohydrates.

This means that your intake of complex, unrefined carbohydrates should be increased at the same time that your intake of simple, refined carbohydrates should be limited and carefully watched. When measured gram for gram, all carbohydrates have the same caloric value; however, different sources of carbohydrates vary in nutritional value. There are three different types of carbohydrates. These are monosaccharides, disaccharides, and polysaccharides. The simple carbohydrate, sugar, is an example of a mono- or disaccharide. Monosaccharides are sugars containing one sugar group per molecule, and disaccharides are sugars containing two sugar groups per molecule. These simple or refined carbohydrates should be limited in your diet.

The complex carbohydrates, the type that should be increased in your diet, are polysaccharides, which contain many sugar groups per molecule. Complex carbohydrates are found in dried beans and peas, grains, and vegetables. The natural sugar found in fruit and milk is an example of a simple carbohydrate. Refer back to chapter 8, "Sweeteners." When these simple carbohydrates are refined and processed into commercial sugars and other sweeteners, they retain their calories, but nutritionally speaking, the calories found in these refined carbohydrates are "empty." As an example, if you were to eat several grams of confectioners' sugar, a refined carbohydrate, you would be taking in calories, but in terms of nutrition, you would be getting very little.

5. Increase consumption of fiber-containing foods.

It is the opinion of many nutritionists, registered dietitians, and diet counselors that the single most important thing you can do for your health is to greatly increase consumption of fiber. Fiber, or roughage, is the portion of a plant that the human digestive system cannot digest. Good sources of fiber include unrefined complex carbohydrates such as fresh vegetables and fruits, whole grains, peas, and beans. See chapter 10, "A Word About Fiber, Fiber, Fiber," for a discussion of fiber.

6. Reduce the intake of sodium and salt.

There has been a lot of controversy concerning high blood pressure and the intake of too much salt. Generally, Americans consume too much salt, and many manufacturers are aware of this fact and have begun to develop products with lowered sodium content. Table salt, approximately 40 percent sodium, is the main source of sodium in the American diet. Convenience foods and fast foods should be watched for their sodium content. Bacon, pickles, canned soups, peanut butter, and salad dressings are notoriously high in sodium content. Read the package labels and choose a product that has been manufactured with low sodium content.

7. Limit the consumption of alcohol to minimum levels, if consumed at all.

Alcohol has almost no nutritional value. It does contain calories, empty calories, that could cause you to skip a meal. If you drink, moderation is the watchword. One or two drinks per day may not harm you if you are an adult. Pregnant women, of course, should not consume alcohol. See chapter 3, "Party Food and Drink."

12

The Importance of Fresh Vegetables and Salads

I am a strong advocate of fresh vegetables and salads. Does this mean I am a vegetarian? No, it doesn't, and even though I believe diabetics should generally eat more like vegetarians, I still maintain that a varied and balanced diet is the best way to go. I do not think it will come as any surprise to most that research indicates our consumption of red meat and meat products is considered too high in America. In the past, the ability to eat a steak every day was the result of hard work and good fortune. Along with the red meat came high fat content, which brought a host of cardiovascular problems. As a result, cardiovascular disease has become this nation's number one killer.

As research has changed our modern-day perspective, it is interesting to note the advocacy of a high vegetable intake by the American Diabetes Association, the American Dietetic Association, the American Heart Association, and the National Cancer Institute. In years past, part of the problem could have been the subtle notion that anyone tending toward a vegetarian diet had to be some sort of kook, and perhaps even un-American. After all, this country takes justifiably great pride in its beef cattle industry, and as we became more affluent, the consumption of beef and rich meat products increased.

The problems causing heart disease are a lot more complex than a diet rich in red meats; however, many experts do agree that our consumption of protein-rich foods, including fatty meat, is too high. Interestingly, it has taken many years to scientifically prove that we must limit our intake of fat and protein. It was not too long ago that many fast-food restaurants made a major turnaround and began using vegetable oil rather than hog lard for deep-frying.

With time and study, learning to eat lean meats — and less meat — fewer fatty foods, less animal lard, more whole grains and fiber, and a lot more fresh fruit and vegetables will certainly improve anyone's diet, and may substantially improve the health of the diabetic. This is not only an educational problem but also a behavioral problem.

I make a ritual out of preparing vegetables and salads. By ritual I mean that I am meticulously compulsive in the preparation of my vegetables. I want them very clean, very fresh, and at the peak of ripeness. This is neglected by some, but learning to become a careful vegetable shopper is almost as important as thoroughly cleaning and preparing them. I also want a very sharp knife so that I can easily cut and prepare my vegetables. Generally, I like to thinly slice them for inclusion in my salad.

One of my favorite salads from the survival days of college and medical school is what I call the Hawaiian Surfer Salad, a salad I lived on during my days in Hawaii. I use one red, ripe tomato, one-half ripe avocado, one peeled cucumber, one carrot, and red-leaf lettuce, all thinly sliced or finely chopped. I also include three or four chunks of cheddar cheese, three or four black olives, and two or three slices of onion. After placing everything in a large salad bowl, I add a can of red salmon (drained), lemon juice, Italian salad dressing, and a small amount of Kraft Catalina French dressing for taste. You will not believe how good this salad can be. Of course, you can substitute tuna for salmon, or fresh grilled salmon for canned salmon if you have it. I like to eat some type of good crisp wheat crackers or toasted seven-grain whole wheat bread along with it. This is not a salad, it is a meal.

One note of caution when preparing to eat a salad: carefully monitor the amount of salad dressing you add. In years past, I consumed a tremendous amount of calories by adding huge quantities of rich salad dressings such as blue cheese dressing, telling myself it was okay since I was eating all those good greens. In truth, the beneficial effects of salad are diminished by adding too much highly caloric, salty, and fat-laden salad dressing. One way to gradually wean yourself from too much salad dressing is to substitute lemon juice for a portion of the dressing you would normally use. I learned this the hard way some years ago when a friend expressed astonishment at my heavy hand with the blue cheese dressing, asking me if I planned to use all my fat exchanges for the week on my one salad. Thanks to him, I wised up, realizing that a salad dressing should dress a salad, not drown it.

Have you ever had a cauliflower salad? That's right, just cauliflower that has been sliced or cut up into florets and to which you have added some low-fat Italian dressing or just vinegar and oil. There are very few calories here except for the dressing you choose. You can do the same with broccoli, cabbage, cucumbers, radishes, or onions.

Chef's salad is another favorite I either make or order at a restaurant. When making a chef's salad at home, you can add as many ingredients as you'd like to suit your taste. I make my own chef's salad by adding my favorite vegetables and some deli turkey meat and low-fat cheese. Try adding ham, chicken, or tuna salad to your chef's salad to create your own specialties.

Most supermarket produce sections have fresh spinach available. There may be sand particles or dirt left in the stems of the spinach leaves, so wash them carefully and make a great salad using the leaves alone or in combination with other vegetables. Many stores also carry prepackaged cabbage that has been thinly sliced for making coleslaw or a quick cabbage salad, which I use when I am in a hurry.

Plan your fresh vegetable purchases to last approximately one week in the refrigerator. Wash leaf lettuce immediately, dry it, and then replace it in the plastic bag it was purchased in, thus keeping it fresh and crisp. The small amount of water left in the bag enters the leaf tissue and helps to keep it fresh.

When eating carrots, remember that they should be limited on your diet because they are high in sugar. Also, beets contain sugar and must be accounted for in order to watch calories. Olives are a fat and, yes, they too must be limited. Try to increase your intake of leafy vegetables and salads on a daily basis. And don't forget the alfalfa sprouts and bamboo shoots.

13

Fruit and Fruit Sugar

Having lived in Hawaii and California for as long as I did, I am no novice when it comes to fruit. My backyard in California had navel and Valencia orange, tangelo, grapefruit, fig, green apple, and peach trees. We also had an orange grove with over six hundred mature Valencia orange trees that produced so much fruit that we had to have one of the big growers pick the fruit for us. Can you imagine a diabetic who loves to eat fruit set loose in my backyard or in the orange grove? I was that diabetic, going from tree to tree with my trusted companion, a Doberman pinscher who loved to eat all the different kinds of fruit as much as I did. When the Valencia oranges became tree ripened, they tasted better than candy, the sugar content was so high. I can still imagine the wonderful sweetness of a California navel orange, so sweet that eating just one skyrocketed my blood sugar into the danger zone. There I was, a total fruit lover, in fruit heaven but with severe insulin-dependent diabetes.

If you are relating to what I am saying here, a good understanding of the nature of fruit sugar is important for you. I knew darn well that one large, ripe navel orange would send my blood sugar over 250 milligrams per deciliter and higher. When I had finished my second navel orange at one sitting and started thinking about a third, how high do you think my blood sugar rose? To a fruit lover, the sheer delight of such fine fruit made the consequences of long-term hyper- glycemia appear far distant and of no immediate concern. But you must be concerned about any item you eat that can produce high blood sugar. I am human just as you are, and the one thing diabetes demands is the mental stamina to engage your strategy and uplift your positive, enthusiastic thinking when you want so desperately to just give in and eat everything you want.

Do you see any difference between the diabetic who loves to eat sweet, sugary candies all the time and the diabetic who loves to eat too much fruit? If the diabetic gets high blood sugar from eating too much candy, what difference is there in the high blood sugar gained by eating too much fruit? High blood sugar is high blood sugar, right? Before you answer this question, think back to our discussion of fruit sugar (fructose) in chapter 8, "Sweeteners." Think about our discussions of quantity and the impact overeating can have on dia- betes.

Because most fruit contains a lot of sugar, it must be managed on your diet. Remember, candy contains refined sugar (sucrose), which will add to your caloric count but is empty in terms of nutritional value. Fruit contains fructose, which is metabolized more slowly, and this sugar, combined with the nutritional value of fiber and vitamins found naturally in the fruit, makes it valuable for the diabetic. Again, quantity is the key watchword. Eat too many high-sugar-containing fruits and you will have high blood sugar. This is why fruit is a controlled item on the diabetic diet.

Some people get confused when it comes to fruit. Fruit is different from candy, they argue, and besides, it is good for you. Although this is basically true, due to the high sugar content in many fruits, you still need to be prudent.

When I was first diagnosed with diabetes and working to under-stand how the diabetic diet works and how to manipulate it, I was in a quandary over honeydew melon. How much could I eat of this melon, I questioned my parents. They were wondering about it also, because they knew honeydew melon is quite sweet. After consulting my dia-betic diet book and exchange list, my mother figured out how much honeydew I was allowed in my exchanges for one meal. It turned out that I could eat only a very small piece according to my fruit allowance for breakfast. I was terribly disappointed. After all, I was used to eating as much melon as I wanted. My father, seeing how distraught I was, consoled me by telling me I could have honeydew for breakfast, lunch, and dinner as my fruit exchange. In this manner, I would get my fill of the melon, just not all at the same time. My mother and father and I had brainstormed through a diabetic meal dilemma. It was really not the same as eating all the melon I wanted at one time, but I did get to eat my share of melon throughout the day.

I think it is clear that a large piece of melon would have meant high blood sugar, while eating a small amount at a time meant stability. On your prescribed diet, you will be allowed a fruit exchange for each meal. It will be up to you to determine which fruit you will choose and how much of it you can eat.

For me, the replacement of a sweet dessert with fruit, especially after a wonderful meal, is a good alternative. Most diabetics are allowed fruit on their diets anyway, so this is a nice way of comple-menting a meal and avoiding the excessive calories and sugar content in most desserts.

You can think up some wonderful fruit combinations that are delightful to eat. One of my favorites is Banana Dynamite. You cut one banana into slices and add a teaspoon of honey. Add lemon juice and top with almonds. Mix together and enjoy. Check your fruit exchanges and go easy on the honey. This is a very easy way of making a banana into something special. Another favorite is mixed fresh fruit compote. You make it with cut-up apple, orange, banana, melon, grapes, and a little lemon juice.

Today, there are so many different exotic fruits you can enjoy — papaya, mango, guava, Asian pears, kiwi, among a myriad of others — that you should never get bored with fruit. The variety of fruit is fantastic at the larger supermarkets. I like to eat organically grown fruit when I can get it. Organically grown fruit is chemical and pesticide free, and although it may cost a little more, the taste is well worth it. Fruit should always be cleaned, or even scrubbed with a brush, before eating. The skins of apples provide fiber and should not be peeled if possible.

As diabetics, we know that a varied diet that includes fruit is good for us. Fruit sugar, fructose, occurs naturally within the fruit and in well-controlled diabetes will cause less of a dramatic rise in the blood sugar than sucrose, or refined table sugar. Fruit sugar does not turn into free glucose because it is either used immediately or stored quickly by the liver as glycogen and thus metabolizes more slowly if your diabetes is under good glycemic control. Fruit is a wonderful thing to enjoy, and if we follow good diabetes practice and common sense, it is an important asset to our good health.

14

Vegetable and Fruit Juices

O ver the years, there has been a lot of discussion concerning the pros and cons of adding vegetable and fruit juices to the diabetic diet. If you drink canned juices, will there be too many preservatives, salt, and other chemical additives that may be dangerous to your health? If you process your own vegetable and fruit juices with a home juicer, will you lose the beneficial effects of the fiber in the process of extracting the juice?

Let us look briefly at some vegetable and fruit juices and their implications for our better health. I think it comes as no surprise to anyone that if you enjoy vegetables, you probably enjoy vegetable juice, and if you enjoy fruit, then you probably enjoy fruit juice. Healthful natural juices compete with the soft drink industry, if not in terms of market share, then certainly in terms of what is good for us.

Think about what comes to your mind when you are thirsty in the middle of the day. Do you first consider going to the refrigerator and having a soft drink? In order to get your can of soda, you may have to brush past a can of vegetable or fruit juice. Why is it that for most of us, the first thing we consider when we are thirsty is a Coke or other carbonated soft drink? Is it the millions of dollars spent on advertising these products that sends you automatically to get a soft drink when you are just the least bit thirsty?

Perhaps this is the modern American way, and we should just give in to the fact that convenience foods and convenience drinks have made our fast-paced lives a little easier. But is this convenience good for us in terms of our health? When was the last time it occurred to you to order a can of vegetable or fruit juice at a fast-food restaurant? Thankfully, some of the fast-food restaurants offer orange juice, but this is usually only for their breakfast menus, as most people would not order it at other times.

Drinking a soft drink may be some sort of by-product of mass programming. Many people feel that a soft drink is the only choice to order with a meal. I was a diet soft drink junkie in years past. I would drink at least two to three diet sodas per day, thus reducing my intake of water. Some of my friends will drink four or more soft drinks per day.

If you find that you may be drinking too many soft drinks, perhaps you could wean yourself off them and try filtered or purified bottled water and vegetable and fruit juices. You may not be able to or even want to give up sodas all at once. Trying to supplement your diet with vegetable and fruit juices and a lot of clean water is, in my opinion, a good way to go.

Canned V-8 vegetable juice is one of my favorites, and I have been drinking it for many years. Let's take a look at what it contains:

V-8 100% Vegetable Juice
Can size: 11.5 fluid ounces
Serving size: 6 fluid ounces
Servings per container: 1.9
Calories: 35
Fat: 0 grams
Protein: 1 gram

Carbohydrates: 8 grams

Cholesterol: 0 mg

Sodium: 490 mg

Potassium: 370 mg

Dietary fiber: 1 gram

Contents: Tomato juice from concentrate (water, tomato concentrate), reconstituted vegetable juices (carrots, celery, beets, parsley, lettuce, watercress, and spinach), salt, vitamin C (ascorbic acid), spice extract, and citric acid

There are two items on the ingredients list that you may want to take note of when you drink V-8 vegetable juice. First, the average serving size of six fluid ounces contains quite a lot of sodium. If you are on a sodium-restricted diet, this may be entirely too much for you. Second, the potassium level is high, for those who must watch their intake of potassium, such as diabetics who are experiencing renal insufficiency. V-8 vegetable juice contains no fat and only thirty-five calories per serving. This is a delightful way to get a gram of dietary fiber and a wonderful combination of vegetables. Remember, watch the sodium and potassium if you are restricted on these items, and if you are unsure, discuss it with your dietitian.

If you like plain tomato juice, you can add a little pepper or Tabasco sauce, lemon, and some Worcestershire sauce and have a fantastic health drink. You need to be careful with carrot juice, as carrots have sugar in them. If you stop in a health food store that has a juice bar, ask them to make you a carrot-celery juice drink. Celery contains salt and will offset the sweetness of the carrot juice, resulting in a fantastic taste you may want more often.

Who can resist a glass of fresh-squeezed orange juice? You know how I feel about fruit, especially oranges, from the chapter on fruit and fruit sugar, so obviously I love fresh-squeezed orange juice. Apple juice, prune juice, and many other fruit juices taste wonderful, but be most cautious and judicious in the amount you drink at one time. These juices are high in sugar content, and because they taste so good, many diabetics will overindulge.

I always keep a supply of fresh orange juice on hand for the treatment of insulin reactions. For myself, I have found orange juice to be one of the quickest-acting "reversers" of hypoglycemia, the insulin reaction. I keep small drink boxes of orange juice in my desk, brief-case, and car, and especially at my bedside, where I may suffer an insulin reaction in the middle of the night or early-morning hours. For those occasional reactions that are more severe, add several table-spoons of pure sugar to the orange juice.

Another juice I find beneficial to my health is cranberry juice. I usually drink about four to eight ounces of cranberry juice every day. Cranberry juice keeps the kidneys and the urinary tract flushed out and may reduce the buildup of crystalline deposits within the delicate structures of the urinary tract. This is a very good and clean-tasting juice that is not especially heavy with sugar. Always buy cranberry juice and any other fruit juice without any added sugar.

There are several good books on the market today that expound upon the good health benefits of some vegetable and fruit juicers. These units are fun to have around if you enjoy making your own vegetable and fruit juices. The juice extractor will literally make juice out of any vegetable or fruit placed in it. The pulp of the vegetable or fruit, where the beneficial fiber is found, is sloughed off and collected into a special chamber for disposal. Some experts have found ways of cooking with this fiber material and use it in sauces and pasta, rice, and meat dishes.

In whatever manner you choose to add vegetable and fruit juices to your diet, they should make an important addition to your diet and provide a great benefit to your overall health.

15

The Role of Family and Friends

*I*n the ideal family situation, when one member becomes sick, the others gather around and offer healing in the form of physical, emotional, and spiritual uplifting. In this way, strength from the larger healthy group is transferred to the sick individual. The rather unknown factors responsible for this exchange are not well understood by modern medical science, but the power it wields can certainly be witnessed. Modern drug therapy, high-tech instrumentation, well-trained doctors, and associated health professionals complement the factors that are expressed through the healing and nurturing of the family unit.

It is my opinion that when a family member is diagnosed with diabetes, other family members must gather around and provide strong emotional and psychological strength and support. In the case of a young child, a very definite sense of confidence and strength must be transmitted in order for the child to feel that everything is under control, even if the parents feel that it is not. In the case of the elderly person diagnosed with diabetes, it is important that depression and a sense of loss do not become overwhelming. Family support can be vitally important here.

When I was first diagnosed with diabetes, my family had no real understanding of the complex nature of this disease. There were horror stories that anyone found to have "sugar diabetes" was sentenced to a shortened life and one that was sure to be filled with complications, pain, and suffering. Once my diagnosis was made, action was taken by my parents to read all the books available on diabetes. I was admitted into the hospital for a week in order to get my disease under control and to learn how to manage it myself. Within this short period of time, we had managed to learn enough about diabetes to be able to "speak the language." Instead of fighting against diabetes, my family loved me enough to realize that, theoretically, we might as well all have had the disease, with me carrying the responsibility of managing the necessary routine on a daily basis.

Some diabetes experts have developed great family involvement strategies over the years. One such strategy that I think is interesting is for the entire family to live as the diabetic must live for one week. This includes injections with sterile saline to all family members at the same time the diabetic must administer his or her own insulin injection. The diet followed by the diabetic is roughly approximated by all family members with avoidance of sugar, sweet desserts, and sugar sodas. A program of exercise is carried out by each family member, just as the diabetic would do. This family group activity, although some critics have labeled it as going too far, helps to create confidence and emotional stability for the diabetic, especially at a time when the diabetic may be experiencing the trauma of feeling as if he or she were the only person on earth having to take insulin injections, learn a new diet regime, and exercise regularly, whether he or she wants to do this or not.

Several years ago, my girlfriend and I planned to meet my younger brother and his girlfriend for dinner at a very fine restaurant. Suzie and I got to the restaurant just prior to the time I usually take my evening insulin injection. The atmosphere in the restaurant was quiet and reserved. When my brother and his girlfriend arrived, we all ordered some wine and began talking. As we relaxed, we began to talk and laugh a little louder. The people around us caught our gaiety and began to talk a little louder and laugh also. Everyone in the restaurant was having a great time, including me, who was probably laughing the most. All of a sudden, Suzie tugged on my arm and insisted we go to the restroom area of the restaurant. I took Suzie's arm so that she could lead me. Still not understanding what she wanted, I asked her what was wrong. "It's you, Joe," she said.

"What do you mean, Suzie?" I asked, feeling guilty but not knowing why. "Joe, you are high as a kite. I bet your blood sugar is over three hundred. You have not taken your insulin yet, and I am worried about you," she said.

Then it dawned on me that I had not taken my insulin injection. With Suzie's help, I tested my blood sugar and found it to be over three hundred milligrams per deciliter, just as Suzie had predicted. I took my insulin and we returned to the table to begin our great dinner.

In this case, Suzie was more in tune with my diabetes than I was. Her intuition that I was getting a little out of control along with her knowledge of diabetes in general, and my case of diabetes in particular, told her I needed to take my insulin injection. I will never forget this incident and her caring attitude and concern for me.

Here is another real-life situation from my past — this time it was a group of friends who came to my rescue. We were all to meet for lunch at the local Mexican restaurant, and as it was twelve noon, the lunch crowd was in full force. We ordered our favorite selections and ate tortilla chips and drank iced tea while we talked and waited for our lunch to be served. Due to the large number of people at the restaurant this day, our meals were greatly delayed. I knew that I was quickly spiraling downward into an insulin reaction but felt that the food must be on its way any moment. My friends continued talking and eating chips as I broke out into a full-body sweat. I became confused and disoriented. I could not say anything to my friends and was not a part of the conversation. My thoughts varied wildly, and I could not put the topic of their conversation into focus. Suddenly, my good friend's wife said, "Hey, why isn't Joe saying anything?"

When I did not respond to this question, she quickly ran to one of the waitresses and asked her to bring a sugar Coke immediately. I drank down the Coke and within a few minutes was able to thank my friend for her help and her realization that I was in a severe insulin reaction.

As the preceding examples demonstrate, your friends and associates should be brought into the diabetes equation also. If they do not know what to do for an insulin reaction, and if you have not prepared them for such an incident, then they will not be able to help you properly if such an incident should occur. Once your friends and associates are informed of your diabetes and how to help in an emergency, they should be only too happy to be of assistance. This is doubly true if you do a good job in describing the grave nature of and quick response that is necessary in treating an insulin reaction.

For the diabetic and his or her family, learning to eat well-balanced, high-carbohydrate, and high-fiber meals with lowered amounts of fat and protein and with the inclusion of fresh vegetables and fruit will greatly enhance the health of all the family members, from youngest to oldest. Learning to adopt some of the healthy ways of life that are so vitally important for the diabetic is only logical good sense for those without diabetes, for it is my opinion that the diabetic's healthy way of life will make a healthy person even healthier. Why not start young children off on the road to good nutrition at the earliest age possible? Good nutritional training at an early age means that good nutrition will become a way of life.

I would like to add only one comment to this discussion of the role of the family and diabetes, and it tends to be part of my personal philosophy. As far as I am concerned, I am the person with diabetes in my family. Just because I cannot eat all the chocolate cake I want, drink all the sugar soft drinks I want, or drink all the beer I want, does not mean that another person without diabetes should not do these things. It is my opinion that they probably should not, but really, this is their decision. It may take you some time to develop your own personal philosophy, but be mindful of the fact that although not everyone is diabetic, they must be as careful with their diets and their lives as you must be.

If you make a habit of always announcing that you cannot eat a certain item or drink a sugar soda because you have diabetes, you may become a terrible bore, and your family and friends may feel somewhat irritated. I think you understand my point here. You are the person with diabetes and the responsibility begins and ends with you. Take this advice for what it is worth to you. I feel that tempering any "eating" situation — whether dining with family or friends at home or at a restaurant — with good common sense, balance, and control is the best way to go.

Once you and your family develop confidence in your ability to manage the challenge that diabetes represents, the daily management skills will become a way of life for you and your family. This attitude will extend to your other relationships — friends and associates, business or otherwise.

And yes, my mother and father still watch over me to see that I do not forget my insulin, that I have plenty to eat, and that I have my late-night snack. Thanks, Mom. Thanks, Dad.

16

Compliance, Diabetes, and a Healthy Life

*A*n editorial commentary by a California physician appearing in a medical journal related the term *sweat equity*, and credited this term to the television show *This Old House*. What he meant by this was patient participation in preventive programs, diet, exercise, and disease education.

I think that this so-called sweat equity can be directly applied to the energy it takes to deal adequately with diabetes and the diabetic diet. The diabetic cannot act as a passive participant in his or her disease, but rather must become totally involved in the "blood, sweat, and tears," hard work, dedication, and discipline that are a part of this sweat equity.

The concept of becoming a healthy diabetic involves more than just eating the correct items and in the correct quantities. Our focus in this book has been directly on the diet therapy within good diabetes management. However, this must include the correct medication protocol and home blood glucose monitoring along with a good exercise program. It will be up to you to develop a program of exercise that is done on a routine basis. In order to become a healthy diabetic, a meticulous program of all three of the major components of the diabetes management regime must be followed carefully, and although we all experience times when we will stray, adherence to this program most of the time is in our best interest.

If you were to poll a group of endocrinologists about one of the biggest problems in dealing with health care to diabetics, many would probably say it is compliance, that is, compliance with the diabetic regime of a healthy diet, a vigorous exercise program, scrupulous monitoring of blood sugars, and meticulous attention to insulin injections or oral medication. This is a tall order. Compliance to every facet of this program requires a great deal of stamina and stick-to-itiveness.

Unfortunately, diabetes does not allow you the luxury of dealing with the disease today but not tomorrow. Diabetes requires close management and attention to detail every day. This program must become a part of your life, automatically instituted on a daily basis. A very dear professor of mine, a diabetologist and endocrinologist, described diabetes as "a ghost disease." He meant that diabetes can go on for years veritably unnoticed, as serious long-term complications may not appear for ten or even twenty years. However, the icy fingers of this ghostlike apparition affix an unmistakably firm grip when the first long-term complication appears.

Take on the attitude that you are in the diabetes business for the long term. Follow your doctors' orders and recommendations, listen attentively as your dietitian plans out a healthy diet for you, and put into daily practice what you learn and study about diabetes. I cannot stress enough how important it is to see your doctor regularly. It will be up to your doctor to determine how often this should be. Also, consultation with your dietitian on a regular basis, at least until you are comfortable with your diabetic diet, is a good idea.

Over the years, I have found it interesting that many diabetics with several years of experience with their disease think they know more about diabetes and the diabetic diet than their doctors. I must own up to the fact that this stupid attitude was my own when I thought I knew all there was to know about diabetes. I had to learn my lesson the hard way, and I hope that you will take my advice and consult with your doctor regularly.

The more a diabetic knows about his or her own disease, the better off that person will be. Knowledge is strength, and as there are many excellent books written on all aspects of diabetes, I urge you to study and read as much as you can. In doing this, your knowledge will dramatically increase as you gain more and more experience in living with diabetes on a daily basis. You will find a selected reading list on pages 388–94.

A diabetic support group may also be helpful for you. In many metropolitan areas the American Diabetes Association sponsors groups where individuals with diabetes gather together to discuss their concerns and possible solutions. I think this is a wonderful way not only to get acquainted with others with diabetes, but also to realize that you are not the only one in the world with this disease. Perhaps your strength may give another diabetic the courage to work harder and thus achieve better health. A more experienced diabetic may be able to offer you support and encouragement when it is your turn to feel a little low. The therapeutic interaction found in these support groups can prove invaluable to you.

Evidence indicates that diabetes has been with us on this planet since before recorded history. Through the millions of man-hours spent studying diabetes, some very good technology has been developed to help us to live with and manage the disease. The disposable syringe comes immediately to mind as does home blood glucose monitoring and nutritional research into the role of soluble and insoluble fiber.

Further technological advances will certainly make diabetes easier to live with in the not too distant future. The near-infrared noninvasive blood glucometer, which requires no finger stick in order to take a blood sample, is just one example. For today, we must continue to strive to normalize our blood glucose through judicious insulin administration or oral antidiabetic medication, vigorous exercise, and meticulous attention to a healthful diet.

Another aspect for the healthy diabetic to consider is the deep relaxation that can be achieved through meditation. This involves attaining a positive state of mind, the cornerstone of my thinking for this book. Using these disciplines, the diabetic can go beyond the traditional thinking of what cannot be done and negative rewards, to that of desire, belief, and expectation of only the most positive rewards and only the best possible outlook for the future. Some researchers are predicting that the application of positive mental power over disease processes of the body may be one of the greatest advances in the history of medicine. But we should remember that this is not new to this century: Aristotle and Socrates told us that the mind could heal the body long ago.

One last area I would like to mention concerns the spiritual. There are many unanswered questions in medicine. I know because I have asked many of these questions and pondered why we do not have answers. I questioned why I became diabetic when I was first diagnosed. When complications of diabetic retinopathy set in and eventually led to total blindness, I asked why such tragedy would happen to me in the prime of my life and career. I renewed my investigations of the insidious nature of diabetic retinopathy and why some diabetics will lose eyesight and others will not. I questioned the total nature of diabetes, the eons of time it has been with us, and again, and many times, why this all had to happen to me.

I urge you to institute a positive-thinking approach to the diabetic diet and living with diabetes. Harness the power of your mind in order to see yourself in perfect health and living well. After all, what do you have to lose?

This is a way of life that involves much more than just diet alone. When I was twenty years old, I achieved a black belt in Shoto Kan, a form of Japanese karate. I had begun studying martial arts at age fourteen in the ninth grade. I believe the rigorous exercise demanded by my early karate instructor was partially responsible for saving my life while I was still an undiagnosed, uncontrolled diabetic. In order to attain the rank of black belt, I had to practice daily for many years, and I began thinking as a martial artist. If we want something badly enough, the level of human tenacity we can develop is amazing.

It is my prayer that you can develop this tenacity for living in a healthy manner with your diabetes.

Introduction to the Recipes

*I*t is with great pride that I introduce to you a fantastic chef and a friend who has put her heart into developing gourmet-class recipes for the diabetic. A diabetic meal plan is a complex, technical, and scientifically formulated regime that enables the diabetic to incorporate a medication schedule and exercise into a balanced program. Because Dianne is not diabetic herself, developing wonderful-tasting meals that must meet a litany of requirements was a tall order for her to fill.

As you review the recipe selections, I believe you will feel as I do that Dianne has created a breakthrough in the traditional thinking of meals planned for the diabetic. Each recipe is a unique creation that meets the specific health challenges faced by the diabetic while also taking into consideration the health of others who may be restricted to low fat intake, low sodium, and low cholesterol. They are, quite simply, fantastic.

— Joe Juliano

When I met Joe Juliano in 1990, I had been cooking professionally both as chef and sous-chef for about fifteen years. He was dining with mutual friends who asked me to prepare something for him that was both sugar free and low in fat but flavorful. I did and he was pleased with my efforts. We began discussing food and found that health and nutrition were common interests.

On that night a collaboration of sorts was born. Whenever we met, our conversation would always come around to food — our attitude toward food, the importance it has in our lives, what we like to eat, what we cannot eat. Finally we began discussing the diabetic's diet and what might be done to make it more flavorful and interesting.

Naturally for food to be all it should be, it has to be delicious as well as heart-healthy, low in fat, and high in fiber content. I like to think of this type of food as "food for the new millennium." This is the way we *all* should eat whether we are diabetic, have heart problems, suffer from hypertension, or just want to be healthy. It is with this idea in mind that Joe and I set about writing our book in the winter of 1992.

The recipes I have come up with reflect what surely will be the dominant trend in food. In my efforts to create these recipes, I had invaluable assistance regarding nutritional information from Carolyn Patterson, a licensed registered dietitian. The nutritional values given at the end of each recipe were calculated per serving.

Enjoy the recipes and use them in good health!

— Dianne Young

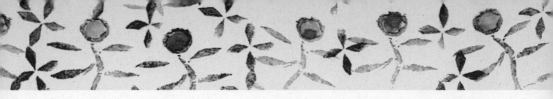

Appetizers

Vegetable Hummus

Texas Pesto

Yogurt and Cucumber Dip

Spinach Dip

Roasted Eggplant Dip

Pita Crisps

Sautéed or Grilled Ginger Tofu
with Teriyaki Sauce

Hot Tofu Salad

Vegetable Rotella

Vegetable Hummus

Hummus is a traditional Middle Eastern appetizer. It is made from pureed chick-peas (garbanzo beans) mixed with tahini (a sesame seed paste similar in consistency to mayonnaise) and served with pita bread. Our version has less fat and fewer calories than the traditional, but it has all of the flavor.

Prepared tahini is fairly high in calories and fats, so I suggest using a dried tahini mix (available in health food stores), which has a lower calorie and fat count. If the dried tahini mix is not easily obtainable, use the tahini that is already mixed or eliminate the tahini completely and substitute a mixture of 2 teaspoons canola oil and 1 teaspoon olive oil.

Remember, if you are using dried chick-peas, you need to either soak the beans overnight or submerge in boiling water for 5 minutes, cover, remove from the heat, and let soak for 1 hour. You must then cook the beans until they are tender (1½ to 2 hours).

1 medium carrot, peeled and thinly sliced

1 small red bell pepper, stemmed, seeded, and julienned

1 celery stalk, sliced into ½-inch pieces

3 tablespoons minced garlic

2 tablespoons minced green onions or scallions (green parts only) or minced fresh chives

2 tablespoons chopped fresh basil, or 1 teaspoon dried

¼ teaspoon cayenne pepper (use less for a less spicy taste)

½ teaspoon salt substitute, optional

1¼ cups cooked chick-peas (about ⅔ cup dried), or 1 (16-ounce) can, drained

2 tablespoons tahini

2 tablespoons fresh lime or lemon juice

1 tablespoon minced fresh parsley

Steam the carrot, bell pepper, and celery in a steamer until tender, about 5 minutes. Thoroughly drain the vegetables and place in a bowl. Add the garlic, green onions, basil, cayenne pepper, and salt substitute, if desired. Let this mixture rest for at least 5 minutes to gather flavor.

Meanwhile, combine the chick-peas, tahini, lime juice, and parsley.

Using either a food processor with a steel blade or a blender, combine the vegetable mixture with the chick-pea mixture and process until smooth. If the hummus is too thick, add water, a few drops at a time, until the desired consistency is reached. Serve with Pita Crisps (page 103).

YIELD: 1½ cups   SERVING SIZE: ¼ cup

Calories	Protein	Carbohydrates	Fat	Sodium
72	3.9 g	12 g	2 g	13 mg

Exchange: 1 starch

Texas Pesto

Unlike traditional pesto, this pesto has no cheese, very few nuts, and very little oil. I make the pesto with either fresh basil or cilantro, depending on what I have in the garden. Both are delicious.

This keeps in the refrigerator for several months and can be used as a dip with Pita Crisps (page 103) or fresh vegetables. Or you may prefer to use it as a condiment with fish, chicken, beans, tacos, or enchiladas. I also like it with plain steamed rice.

3 cups fresh basil or cilantro leaves
¼ to ½ cup sliced pickled jalapeño
*   peppers and some of their*
*   pickling vinegar*
2 tablespoons blanched sliced
*   almonds*

2 teaspoons white wine vinegar
2 to 4 tablespoons fresh lime or
*   lemon juice*
2 tablespoons extra-virgin olive
*   oil*

Put all of the ingredients in a blender and process until they are thoroughly blended.

Taste and correct the seasoning. Serve.

YIELD: About 2 cups   SERVING SIZE: 2 tablespoons

Calories	Protein	Carbohydrates	Fat	Sodium
9.27	0.53 g	1.08 g	0.81 g	113.95 mg

Exchange: Free

Yogurt and Cucumber Dip

Quick and easy to put together, this is the perfect dip to have on hand when you have a party or want something a little special before dinner. It does need to be refrigerated for at least 45 minutes for the flavor to develop. Serve with jicama sticks, Pita Crisps, or any fresh vegetable.

1 large cucumber, peeled, seeded, and shredded

1 cup plain nonfat yogurt

2 tablespoons minced fresh parsley

1 tablespoon minced fresh dill, or 1 teaspoon dried

2 large garlic cloves, minced

1 tablespoon fresh lime or lemon juice

Coarsely ground black pepper to taste

Jicama sticks, Pita Crisps (page 103), or any fresh vegetable for dipping

Combine all of the ingredients in a medium bowl. Cover and refrigerate for at least 45 minutes. Serve.

YIELD: 1¾ to 2 cups   SERVING SIZE: 3 to 4 tablespoons

Calories	Protein	Carbohydrates	Fat	Sodium
20	1.66 g	3.56 g	0.07 g	21.38 mg

Exchange: ¼ vegetable

Spinach Dip

Make sure that the spinach is really clean. After washing it well in cold water and tearing off the heavy stems, thoroughly drain and spin dry in a salad spinner or squeeze dry with paper towels.

You can easily double or triple this recipe.

½ pound fresh spinach, thoroughly washed, stemmed, and drained

¼ cup chopped fresh parsley

½ cup finely chopped green onions or scallions

½ cup plain nonfat yogurt

½ cup sour cream substitute

¼ teaspoon granulated garlic or garlic powder

½ teaspoon dried dill, crushed

Dash of salt substitute, optional

1 tablespoon fresh lime or lemon juice

Be sure that the spinach is thoroughly dry.

Thinly slice the spinach or quickly pulse it in a food processor for 8 to 10 seconds. Transfer the spinach to a large bowl and mix in the parsley and green onions.

Whisk together the yogurt and sour cream substitute, then beat in the granulated garlic, dill, salt substitute, if desired, and lime juice. Add this to the vegetable mixture; cover and chill. The dip may be refrigerated for up to 24 hours. Serve with Pita Crisps (page 103).

YIELD: 2 cups   SERVING SIZE: 4 to 5 tablespoons

Calories	Protein	Carbohydrates	Fat	Sodium
40	1.4 g	2.4 g	3 g	40 mg

Exchange: ½ vegetable; ½ fat

Roasted Eggplant Dip

This dip may be served at room temperature or chilled. I usually prepare it the day before and serve it chilled. It will keep in the refrigerator for 4 to 5 days. Serve it with jicama sticks, Pita Crisps, or any fresh vegetable.

1 medium eggplant, halved
  lengthwise
3 large ripe plum tomatoes,
  halved
1 medium yellow onion, quartered
5 large garlic cloves, unpeeled
8 large mushrooms, halved
1 medium red bell pepper, stemmed,
  halved, and seeded
½ teaspoon dried thyme, crumbled
1 teaspoon dried basil, crumbled

1 teaspoon dried oregano, crumbled
Coarsely ground black pepper to
  taste
2 tablespoons olive oil
1 tablespoon fresh lime or lemon
  juice
Minced fresh parsley for garnish,
  optional
Jicama sticks, Pita Crisps (page
  103), or fresh vegetables for
  dipping

Preheat the oven to 400°F.

Place the eggplant, cut side down, in a large roasting pan. Place the tomatoes, onion, garlic, mushrooms, and bell pepper on top of and around the eggplant. Sprinkle the herbs and black pepper and drizzle the oil evenly over the vegetables. Bake until tender (about 45 minutes). The eggplant is tender when it can easily be pierced with a knife.

Cool and peel the eggplant and garlic. Place them in the bowl of a food processor with a steel blade and add the rest of the vegetables and any liquid. Add the lime juice and puree until the mixture is very smooth. Turn it out into a bowl and garnish with fresh minced parsley, if desired, or chill for future use.

YIELD: About 4 cups   SERVING SIZE: ¼ cup (4 tablespoons)

Calories	Protein	Carbohydrates	Fat	Sodium
37.83	0.91 g	3.97 g	2.55 g	76.5 mg

Exchange: ½ vegetable; ½ fat

Pita Crisps

These crisps can be used just like crackers or chips. They can be served with any dip or pâté. They are quick to make and if kept in an airtight container will hold for 4 to 5 days easily.

¼ teaspoon dried oregano, crumbled
⅛ teaspoon dried thyme, crumbled
3 whole wheat pita bread rounds
2 teaspoons canola oil

Preheat the oven to 350°F.
Combine the oregano and thyme.

Brush each pita round with the oil and cut into 8 wedges. Place the wedges on a dry cookie sheet and sprinkle with the herb mixture. Bake for about 5 minutes. Turn over and bake 2 minutes more.

YIELD: 24 crisps   SERVING SIZE: 4 crisps

Calories	Protein	Carbohydrates	Fat	Sodium
96	3 g	17 g	2 g	169 mg

Exchange: 1 starch; ½ fat

Sautéed or Grilled Ginger Tofu with Teriyaki Sauce

This is a quick and easy appetizer to serve when you have last-minute guests or when you want a snack in the middle of the afternoon. Tofu is the Japanese word for the high-protein, low-calorie bean curd that is a very old staple ingredient in both Japanese and Chinese cuisines. It is made from dried soybeans (soya beans). It is bland-tasting and filling and its uses are infinite. It is an excellent, economical protein extender and is now sold in supermarkets as well as Asian markets and health food stores.

This recipe calls for teriyaki sauce, which you can easily make. The recipe I include here is the tastiest sauce I can think of. If you decide to buy the teriyaki, be sure to buy the low-sodium variety.

Teriyaki is traditionally thought of as being Hawaiian, although many insist that it is Japanese in origin. It is delicious whether used as a sauce or as a marinade. Allow at least 1 hour for the tofu to marinate in the sauce.

Grilled Ginger Tofu

½ cup Teriyaki Sauce (recipe
  follows)
½-inch piece fresh ginger, peeled and
  finely minced or grated
3 green onions or scallions, finely
  minced

1 (16-ounce) package extra-firm
  tofu, sliced lengthwise into ½-
  inch-thick pieces
Nonstick cooking spray for
  sautéing

Combine the teriyaki sauce, ginger, and green onions.

Put the tofu slices in a large shallow stainless steel or glass baking dish and pour the teriyaki mixture over them. Turn the tofu every 20 minutes or so for at least an hour or for as long as 2 hours. Drain.

Heat a heavy skillet over high heat, coat it lightly with the cooking spray, and sauté the tofu slices for about 3 minutes on each side, or until thoroughly heated through. Or, if you wish to grill the tofu, grill over medium-hot coals for about 4 minutes on each side, until the desired temperature is reached.

Cut into large cubes and serve.

YIELD: 4 servings   SERVING SIZE: 4 ounces

Teriyaki Sauce

2 tablespoons finely minced fresh
    ginger, or 2 teaspoons ground
3 garlic cloves, finely minced
1 tablespoon dehydrated onion or
    onion flakes

1½ tablespoons brown sugar
    substitute
1 cup reduced- or low-sodium soy
    sauce
6 tablespoons dry sherry

Whisk together the ginger, garlic, onion, brown sugar substitute, soy sauce, and sherry. It will last stored in a jar in the refrigerator for several months. Use as needed.

YIELD: 1¾ cups

Calories	Protein	Carbohydrates	Fat	Sodium
115	12 g	4 g	7 g	186 mg

Exchange: 1½ medium-fat meat; ½ vegetable

Hot Tofu Salad

I normally use this dish as an appetizer, but it would work equally well as a salad. Increase the size of the serving and serve with several vegetable dishes for a complete meal.

Nonstick cooking spray for sautéing
½ pound tofu, cut into ½-inch cubes
3 tablespoons crushed toasted
* sesame seeds*
1 teaspoon dry sherry
3 tablespoons reduced- or low-
* sodium soy sauce*

½ teaspoon sesame oil
3 cups leafy greens (romaine,
* spinach, arugula), washed,*
* drained, and cut into thin*
* ribbons*
¼ cup chopped fresh cilantro
* leaves*

Heat a large (10-inch), heavy-bottomed skillet over medium heat, coat it lightly with the cooking spray, and sauté the tofu for 3 to 4 minutes.

Quickly add the sesame seeds, sherry, soy sauce, and sesame oil. Gently stir the tofu and the dressing mixture for 1 minute.

Fold in the greens, being sure to coat them with the dressing. Cook until heated through. Sprinkle the cilantro over all and serve.

YIELD: 6 servings   SERVING SIZE: ⅔ cup

Calories	Protein	Carbohydrates	Fat	Sodium
59	15 g	3 g	4 g	356 mg

Exchange: ½ medium-fat meat; 1 vegetable

Vegetable Rotella

Rotellas are sheets of fresh pasta filled with sautéed vegetables, rolled up like jelly rolls, wrapped in cheesecloth, and poached for about 20 minutes in boiling water, then drained and chilled. They are fabulous to use as an appetizer and are fairly quick to make. I usually make them the night before I plan to serve them so that they can chill all day in the refrigerator. Sheets of fresh pasta are sold in Italian specialty stores; each 8-by-8-inch sheet weighs 4 ounces. I stuff these with an eggplant filling, but they can be filled with many things — ricotta and spinach, for example.

Nonstick cooking spray for sautéing

1 small eggplant, cut into ½-inch cubes

1 small yellow onion, finely diced

1 small red bell pepper, stemmed, seeded, and finely diced

3 or 4 medium mushrooms, thinly sliced

1 teaspoon dried basil, crumbled

1 teaspoon dried oregano, crumbled

Coarsely ground black pepper to taste

1 (14-ounce) can low-sodium whole peeled plum tomatoes, coarsely chopped, with their juice

1 tablespoon balsamic vinegar

1 tablespoon dry red wine

1 teaspoon granulated sugar substitute

2 (8-by-8-inch) sheets fresh pasta (use any combination — garlic and basil pasta, tomato pasta, red pepper pasta, or plain)

About 1 yard cheesecloth cut into 2 equal pieces

Nonfat, sugar-free Italian salad dressing for serving, optional

Heat a large 10- or 12-inch skillet over medium heat and coat it lightly with the nonstick cooking spray. Put in the eggplant, onion, bell pepper, mushrooms, basil, oregano, and black pepper. Sauté for a few minutes, until the eggplant and the onion begin to soften.

Add the tomatoes and their liquid, vinegar, red wine, and sugar substitute. Simmer the mixture for 10 to 12 minutes. Remove from the heat and let cool.

Meanwhile, bring a gallon of water to a boil in a large roasting or poaching pan (large enough to hold two 8-inch-long rolls that are each about 3 to 4 inches in diameter). When the water begins boiling, turn down the heat so that there is a low boil. Be sure to keep the water volume to a gallon by adding more water if necessary.

Lay one sheet of pasta flat on your work surface. Evenly spread half of the eggplant sauté over the surface of the pasta, leaving ½ inch bare at the bottom and the top of the sheet. Very carefully and as tightly as you can, roll up the pasta with the eggplant sauté inside. When you are done, it should resemble a long jelly roll. Repeat with the other sheet of pasta.

Take one length of cheescloth and roll up one of the rotellas in it. Tie the ends either with string or with strips of the cheesecloth. Repeat with the other rotella.

Drop both rotellas into the gently boiling water and boil them for about 20 minutes. You can tell when they are done, as they will feel very firm when touched with a fork.

Drain the rotellas in the sink or on a rack and let cool to room temperature. I usually wring out the ends that were tied to make sure that the excess water is gone.

Wrap them in plastic wrap and put them in the refrigerator to chill.

The next day, remove the plastic wrap, unroll the cheesecloth, and discard. With a very sharp knife, slice the rotellas into ¾-inch slices and arrange on a plate. Serve them plain or with nonfat, sugar-free Italian salad dressing on the side.

YIELD: 2 rotellas; 20 to 21 (¾-inch) slices

SERVING SIZE: 2 slices

Calories	Protein	Carbohydrates	Fat	Sodium
85	3 g	16 g	1 g	66 mg

Exchange: 1 starch

Breakfast

Cottage Cheese Muffins

Cottage Cheese Pancakes I

Cottage Cheese Pancakes II

German Apple Pancake

Basic Omelet Recipe and Fillings

Cottage Cheese Muffins

These muffins are delicious at breakfast plain or with sugarless jam and are also a great after-school snack with fruit.

Nonstick cooking spray for the
    muffin-pan cups
½ cup whole wheat flour
1 cup unbleached white flour
½ teaspoon salt
2 teaspoons baking powder
The equivalent of 2 eggs in egg
    substitute

1 cup 1% or other very low fat
    cottage cheese
½ teaspoon grated lemon zest
1 teaspoon fresh lemon juice
2 tablespoons low-fat margarine,
    melted
2 tablespoons honey

Preheat the oven to 400°F. Lightly coat 12 muffin-pan cups with the nonstick cooking spray.

In a large bowl, mix the whole wheat flour, white flour, salt, and baking powder.

In a small bowl, combine the egg substitute, cottage cheese, lemon zest and juice, margarine, and honey.

Pour the moist ingredients into the flour mixture, stirring only to combine. Do not overmix.

Spoon the batter into the prepared muffin-pan cups and bake for

17 to 20 minutes. The muffins should be lightly browned. Cool for 5 minutes and remove from the pan.

YIELD: 12 muffins   SERVING SIZE: 1 muffin

Calories	Protein	Carbohydrates	Fat	Sodium
85	3.6 g	14 g	1.5 g	169 mg

Exchange: 1 starch

Cottage Cheese Pancakes I

Griddle cakes, flapjacks, pancakes, and crepes are all really forms of dropped scones. They are small, fairly flat cakes cooked on an oiled skillet or griddle until golden on both sides. They are made from a thick batter and contain a raising agent and are traditionally served warm with butter, jam, or honey.

Our pancakes are not full of fat, are not drenched in butter or laden with high-calorie, high-sugar jams or syrups, and do not have a raising agent, but nothing is lost in the taste department. They are a quick and easy solution for times when you want to serve something a little bit different and need to make a meal when you have next to nothing in the house.

These cottage cheese pancakes work quite well at breakfast or brunch, covered with sugarless syrup or fresh fruit, or they can be part of the evening meal.

1 cup 1% or other very low fat
*   cottage cheese*
The equivalent of 4 eggs in egg
*   substitute*
½ teaspoon vanilla extract

½ cup unbleached white flour
¼ teaspoon salt
Nonstick cooking spray for the
*   griddle*

Put the cottage cheese, egg substitute, vanilla, flour, and salt in a blender and blend until the mixture is absolutely smooth. The batter must be smooth in order to cook properly.

Heat a griddle, large cast-iron skillet, or electric griddle until it is very hot. A drop of water should sizzle when it is flicked onto the griddle. Lightly coat with the nonstick cooking spray.

Pour ¼ to ⅓ cup of the batter onto the griddle for each pancake.

When the surface of the pancakes starts to look dry and stops bubbling, carefully flip the pancakes over and cook for 45 seconds to 1 minute more.

Serve with warmed sugarless jam or cover with fresh fruit.

YIELD: 6 to 8 pancakes   SERVING SIZE: 2 pancakes

Calories	Protein	Carbohydrates	Fat	Sodium
86	8 g	10 g	0.4 g	101 mg

Exchange: 1 lean meat; ½ starch

Cottage Cheese Pancakes II

These cottage cheese pancakes need to cook a little bit longer than "regular" griddle cakes and should be handled gently while you are cooking them.

*The equivalent of 2 eggs in egg
 substitute*
*1 cup 1% or other very low fat
 small-curd cottage cheese*
⅓ cup unbleached white flour
*1 tablespoon granulated sugar
 substitute*

½ teaspoon salt
Dash of ground cinnamon
Dash of ground nutmeg
3 egg whites
⅛ teaspoon cream of tartar
*Nonstick cooking spray for the
 griddle*

In a large bowl, beat together the egg substitute, cottage cheese, flour, sugar substitute, salt, cinnamon, and nutmeg.

In a small bowl, beat the egg whites with the cream of tartar until they are stiff but not dry. Gently fold the beaten whites into the cottage cheese mixture.

Heat a griddle, large cast-iron skillet, or electric griddle until a drop of water sizzles when flicked onto the cooking surface. Lightly coat with the nonstick cooking spray. Pour the batter by ¼ cupfuls onto the griddle.

Cook the pancakes until they are puffy and golden brown on both sides. Top right away with 3 tablespoons fresh fruit, 1 tablespoon apple butter or sugarless syrup, or 2 teaspoons sifted confectioners' sugar substitute, and serve.

YIELD: 12 to 13 pancakes   SERVING SIZE: 2 pancakes

Calories	Protein	Carbohydrates	Fat	Sodium
74	6 g	8 g	2 g	104 mg

Exchange: ½ medium-fat meat

German Apple Pancake

This is one large pancake that is made with grated apples and served with an apple filling. It is high in fiber, low in fat and sugar, and very inexpensive in the winter when fruit can be pricey. It works nicely for breakfast, dinner, or dessert.

The filling can be made in advance and kept in the refrigerator for up to 2 days. Reheat before serving.

Pancake

The equivalent of 3 eggs in egg substitute

¾ cup skim milk

1 teaspoon vanilla extract

¾ cup unbleached white flour

¼ teaspoon salt

1½ tablespoons low-fat margarine

2 teaspoons grated lemon zest

½ cup grated unpeeled apple (Pippin, Newton, Gala, or Granny Smith)

Nonstick cooking spray for the skillet

Filling

¼ cup unsweetened natural apple
  juice
1 tablespoon fresh lemon
  juice
4 to 5 apples, peeled and thinly
  sliced

2 teaspoons granulated sugar
  substitute
½ teaspoon ground cinnamon
½ teaspoon ground nutmeg
Confectioners' sugar substitute for
  topping, optional

Preheat the oven to 450°F.

Prepare the pancake: In a large bowl, beat together the egg substitute, milk, vanilla, flour, salt, margarine, and lemon zest until the mixture is very smooth. Stir in the grated apple.

Heat a large (12-inch), heavy-bottomed ovenproof skillet on the stovetop until quite hot and lightly coat it with the nonstick cooking spray. Pour in the pancake batter and bake in the oven for about 15 minutes. Check during the first 10 minutes or so of baking to make sure that no big bubbles come to the surface of the pancake. If they do, pierce the bubbles with a fork.

After 15 minutes, lower the oven temperature to 350°F and bake for an additional 10 minutes. The pancake will be golden brown and quite crisp when done.

Meanwhile, prepare the filling: Heat the apple juice and lemon juice in a medium saucepan over low heat and add the apples and sugar substitute. Stir, then add the cinnamon and nutmeg. Cover and let simmer for about 10 minutes. The apples should be tender-crisp. This may be done in advance (see headnote).

When the pancake is done, slide it onto a serving platter. Pour the filling onto one side of the pancake and fold the other side over. Top with sifted confectioners' sugar substitute, if desired. Cut the pancake crosswise into 6 slices and serve.

YIELD: 6 servings   SERVING SIZE: 1 (2-inch) slice

Calories	Protein	Carbohydrates	Fat	Sodium
136	3 g	27 g	1.6 g	88 mg

Exchange: 1 starch; 1 fruit

Basic Omelet Recipe and Fillings

Normally, the problem with having eggs for breakfast is the large amount of cholesterol they contain. I mean *real* eggs, not egg substitutes. Technology has now given us a new egg that, theoretically, if used in combination with a low-fat diet, will not make your cholesterol count soar, or even rise, even if you eat as many as 12 per week. Indeed, that is a great innovation and a big help, but I would rather save those new high-tech eggs for poached, soft-boiled, hard-boiled, or basted eggs.

An omelet need not be made with either a whole egg or an egg substitute. For quite some time, I have been preparing omelets with egg whites both at home and professionally and the results have been very successful. Save your egg yolks for something else, or for someone else.

To separate an egg you first need 3 small bowls. Crack open the egg on the side of one of the bowls and immediately put the contents (the yolk and the white) in your hand and let the white run through your fingers into the bowl. Place the yolk in another bowl. Now transfer the separated egg white into the third bowl. Repeat the process, separating the egg over an empty bowl each time, and then transferring the yolks to the bowl where you have the other yolks and the whites to the bowl where you have the other whites. This helps ensure that you get no egg yolk in the egg whites and vice versa. Use the egg whites and either save the yolks or throw them away.

I always use ice water when I make omelets or scrambled eggs, as cold water really helps to make the eggs fluffy and adds no extra fat or calories. Put about 6 ice cubes in a 1-cup measuring cup and fill the cup with water. Stir for a moment then take out the necessary amount of ice water.

2 tablespoons ice water
3 egg whites (for a 2-egg omelet)
Coarsely ground black pepper to taste

Dash of granulated garlic or garlic powder, optional
Dash of salt, optional
Nonstick cooking spray for the pan

With a whisk, beat the ice water into the egg whites. Add the pepper, granulated garlic, and salt, if desired. Whisk again.

Heat a medium (6- or 8-inch) nonstick sauté pan over medium heat. Lightly coat the pan with the nonstick cooking spray and just as soon as the pan is hot enough, add the egg mixture. Using a flexible rubber spatula, gently lift the edges of the omelet as it begins to set and allow all of the egg that is still liquid to flow underneath the "set" egg and cook.

Add whatever filling you wish (see page 122 for some suggestions), put a lid on the sauté pan, and allow the omelet to finish cooking and the filling to heat through, about 1½ minutes.

When the omelet is done, slide it from the pan onto a plate and fold it with the edge of the pan or with a spatula. Serve immediately.

If serving more than 1 person, either use a larger pan and cut the omelet in half or make the omelets one at a time and hold them in a

225°F oven until all are done. The eggs will keep nicely for 6 to 7 minutes.

YIELD: 1 omelet

Calories	Protein	Carbohydrates	Fat	Sodium
45	9 g	0 g	0 g	150 mg

Exchange: 1 lean meat

Fillings

When you are going to serve filled omelets, you will make your job easy and fast by preparing the filling ingredients ahead of time. This means the cheese should be grated, the onion diced, the mushrooms, potatoes, and bell peppers precooked, and the spinach washed and stemmed. Precooking the vegetables does not affect the quality of the dish; the vegetables will heat up immediately when they are added to the surface of the eggs and the pan is covered. By having everything ready to go, you can easily entertain at breakfast or brunch or simply feed your family their favorite omelet or let them make their own from the assembled ingredients.

SOME FILLING SUGGESTIONS

1. Combine ¼ cup chopped fresh spinach; 2 large mushrooms cut into thin slices and sautéed; 1 tablespoon finely diced onion sautéed with a bit of minced fresh garlic; and a dash of fresh Parmesan cheese.

2. Combine ¼ cup red and green bell pepper slices, sautéed; 1 tablespoon finely diced onion sautéed with a bit of minced fresh garlic; and 1 small tomato, diced, tossed with a pinch of oregano and basil and some grated Parmesan cheese. Top the filled omelet with heated Marinara Sauce (page 171) if you wish.

3. Combine 3 tablespoons cooked, shredded chicken; thinly sliced yellow corn tortilla strips; 2 teaspoons sliced green chilies; 1 tablespoon finely diced onion sautéed with a bit of minced fresh garlic; ½ small tomato, diced; and a dash of ground cumin in a dry skillet and heat for about 1 minute. Sprinkle with 2 tablespoons shredded Monterey Jack cheese after turning the mixture onto the eggs.

4. Combine 1 small red potato, steamed and diced; ½ small carrot cut into julienne strips and steamed; ¼ cup sautéed thin-sliced red cabbage; 1 tablespoon plain nonfat yogurt; a dash of crumbled dried dill; a pinch of crushed caraway seeds; and a splash of fresh lime juice.

Broths and Soups

A Word About Soup

Vegetable Broth

Potato Peel Broth

Garlic Broth

Chicken Broth

Beef Broth

Simple Noodle Soup

Spinach Soup

Winter Green Soup

Beet-Top Borscht

Chilled Blender Borscht

Onion Soup

Minestrone

Carrot and Sweet Potato Soup

Spicy Corn-and-Tortilla Soup

Lime-Tarragon French Fish Soup (Pot-au-Feu)

Northwest Cioppino

Mulligatawny Soup (Stew)

A Word About Soup

Any hearty soup can easily serve as an entrée, and when put together with the proper proteins, side dishes, salads, and breads, can help form a completely nutritious meal. A satisfying meal should be balanced in its variety of dishes, in much the same way a really good recipe is balanced in its use of ingredients. Think of your whole meal as one recipe, with each dish as an ingredient in that recipe. The easiest way of achieving this literally is with soup. It's nutritious and has a myriad of flavors tied together with the broth or stock. The liquid may have a few extra calories, but it allows you to have small amounts of things you normally might not eat, such as shrimp, sausage, bacon, and butter. The broth carries the flavor of those high-fat items, which is what you crave, without your having to have a big serving of something loaded with animal fat to get it. Food should be good for you, and eating should be both pleasurable and immediately gratifying. But if you are on a restricted diet, it is often hard to see food as anything other than the enemy. Soups can help bridge the gap between what you know you should eat and what you want to eat.

Soups are also great time-savers when cooking. The broth can be made in advance and frozen until needed. Soups can be put together very quickly, which is a real boon in the workaday world when there are not hours set aside in one's time budget for cooking.

Vegetable Broth

This broth and the following vegetable broths are delicious served on their own, but they are also tremendously useful for making other soups and sauces. (Please note, in my cooking broths and stocks are the same; both can stand alone as a nutritious soup or as a base for other soups.)

The carrots and the celery give a light sweetness to the broth, while the mushrooms and the potatoes give it strength.

This broth may be kept in the refrigerator for 3 to 4 days and can be frozen for 3 to 4 months.

3 medium celery stalks with their leaves, cut into chunks

2 medium onions, unpeeled and stuck with 2 whole cloves each

4 to 5 garlic cloves, unpeeled and lightly crushed

2 medium potatoes, thoroughly scrubbed and cut into large chunks

4 to 5 large carrots, peeled and cut into large chunks

10 large brown cremini or primavera mushrooms, halved

1 large leek, white end trimmed, split in half lengthwise, and thoroughly washed, rinsed, and cut in half (see Note, page 154)

2 ripe medium tomatoes, cut in half

6 large sprigs of fresh parsley

Large pinch of dried thyme, crumbled

Large pinch of dried oregano, crumbled

3 large bay leaves, crumbled

12 whole black peppercorns

2 teaspoons salt

4 quarts cold water

Combine all of the ingredients in a large, heavy pot. Bring to a boil over high heat, lower the heat, and simmer, uncovered, for about 1 hour. Taste and correct the seasoning.

Simmer for 30 to 45 minutes more. The broth is done when the flavor is full and strong.

Strain the broth through a colander and again through a fine-meshed strainer. Discard the cooked vegetables.

Cool to room temperature and refrigerate or freeze.

YIELD: 8 cups   SERVING SIZE: ⅔ cup if used
                                                         as a soup

Calories	Protein	Carbohydrates	Fat	Sodium
49	1.3 g	10.93 g	0 g	22 mg

Exchange: 2 vegetables

Potato Peel Broth

This recipe is a heartier alternative to the preceding vegetable broth recipe and can be used in any soup recipe. It is also delicious on its own. Rather than worrying about trying to accumulate enough potato peels at one time to make the broth, every time I peel potatoes, I toss the peels in a Ziploc bag and save them in the freezer. Then when I have about 3 cups of potato peels, I make the broth.

For this broth, I use brown-skinned potatoes and cut away any blemishes if necessary.

¼-inch-thick peels from 7 or 8 well-scrubbed large potatoes

1 large onion, unpeeled and cut into quarters

3 large carrots, peeled and cut into large chunks

3 medium celery stalks with their leaves

10 cups cold water

3 large sprigs of fresh parsley

2 small bay leaves

Large pinch of dried thyme, crumbled

Large pinch of dried oregano, crumbled

1 teaspoon salt

10 to 12 whole black peppercorns

4 garlic cloves, unpeeled and lightly crushed

2 tablespoons fresh lime or lemon juice

Combine all of the ingredients except for the lime juice in a large, heavy pot. Bring to a boil over high heat and then lower the heat and simmer, uncovered, for about 1½ hours.

Take care that the liquid does not evaporate too much during the simmering process, and if it does, add more water to keep the vegetables covered. At this point all of the vegetables should be very soft and almost mushy. Taste and correct the seasoning.

The broth should be light brown in color, very fragrant, and delicious. If the taste is too weak, simmer the broth a bit longer to reduce the liquid, which will intensify the taste.

Stir in the lime juice at the very end of the cooking.

Strain the broth through a fine-meshed strainer. Press the vegetables through the mesh with the bottom of a large spoon until only dry pulp is left. This will give you a thicker broth with a slurry texture. If a clear broth is desired, strain it through a fine-meshed strainer but do not push the vegetables through.

Cool to room temperature and refrigerate or freeze.

YIELD: *7* cups

SERVING SIZE: ⅔ cup if used as a soup

Calories	Protein	Carbohydrates	Fat	Sodium
22	0.83 g	5 g	0 g	13 mg

Exchange: 1 vegetable

Garlic Broth

This broth is a delicious addition to your vegetarian broth recipes. It is so clear and visually pleasing that you will want to use it often in soups or any recipe that calls for a stock. Its refrigerated shelf life is the same as that of any vegetable broth, 3 to 4 days, or it can be frozen.

3 medium potatoes, thoroughly
    scrubbed and cut into quarters
1 large onion, unpeeled and halved
    lengthwise
2 large carrots, peeled
2 large celery stalks with their
    leaves
10 cups cold water
2 large sprigs of fresh parsley
2 teaspoons extra-virgin olive oil

1 large bay leaf, crumbled
Large pinch of dried thyme,
    crumbled
1 teaspoon salt
8 whole black peppercorns
3 large heads of garlic, broken
    up into cloves and left
    unpeeled
1 tablespoon fresh lime or lemon
    juice

Combine all of the ingredients except for the lime juice in a large, heavy pot. Bring to a boil over high heat, lower the heat, and simmer, uncovered, for about 1½ to 2 hours.

As with any broth or stock, if too much liquid evaporates during the simmering process, be sure to add more water to keep the vegetables covered.

Taste and correct the seasoning. If the broth is fragrant and tasty, it is done. If not, simmer a bit longer. Stir in the lime juice and strain through a fine-meshed strainer. Cool to room temperature and refrigerate or freeze.

YIELD: 7 cups

SERVING SIZE: ⅔ cup if used as a soup

Calories	Protein	Carbohydrates	Fat	Sodium
40	0.86 g	8 g	0.66 g	10 mg

Exchange: ½ starch

Chicken Broth

You cannot make a good sauce or soup without using a good broth as your base. You can buy low-fat or low-sodium broths in the supermarket, but if you make them yourself you can give them whatever flavor you want through the use of herbs and you can better control the amount of fat. Homemade broths are also far less expensive.

You can use chicken or turkey bones alone, or you can also mix skinned and defatted chicken or turkey pieces in with the bones. I like to get chicken breast "frames" from my butcher. The breast frames are the bones left after the skinless, boneless chicken breasts have been prepared. They produce a really flavorful broth and help to minimize the fat. You might talk to your supermarket butcher to see if there are chicken bones available for sale.

To help ensure that I remove all the fat I possibly can, I put the broth in the refrigerator for 6 to 12 hours after I have strained and cooled it. I can then easily see and remove all of the congealed fat from the top of the broth. The broth can be held for 3 to 4 days in the refrigerator, or frozen for 3 to 4 months.

Often I make my broth in a Crock-Pot (slow cooker), putting all the ingredients in the pot in the morning before I go to work and straining it when I come home.

About 2 pounds chicken or turkey
bones (see headnote)
1½ gallons cold water
2 large yellow onions, unpeeled and
quartered (onion skins give the
broth a bit more flavor and a
beautiful golden color)
3 large carrots, peeled

2 large celery stalks with their
leaves
3 large bay leaves
2 tablespoons whole black
peppercorns
6 large sprigs of fresh parsley
, 1 teaspoon salt, optional
4 garlic cloves, unpeeled

Put the chicken bones and water in a large, heavy pot. Add the remaining ingredients and bring to a boil over high heat. Lower the heat, partially cover, and simmer for 2½ to 3 hours. Add water as needed to maintain the volume. Taste and correct the seasoning. If a stronger flavor is desired, cook for another hour. When the broth is done, remove the bones and vegetables and discard. Strain the broth into a container, cool to room temperature, and refrigerate for several hours. Skim the congealed fat from the surface of the broth.

Keep the broth refrigerated or freeze it for future use.

YIELD: 1 gallon (16 cups)   SERVING SIZE: 1 cup if used as a soup

Calories	Protein	Carbohydrates	Fat	Sodium
11.56	0.31 g	2.50 g	0 g	9.56 mg

Exchange: Free

Beef Broth

Beef broth can be a really welcome addition to soups and sauces. I always use it when making Onion Soup (page 145), but it also works well served on its own.

I use veal bones (which you can get from your butcher) along with beef shank or soup bones. This combination produces a more flavorful broth and also helps cut down on the fat content. Have your butcher crack the veal bones, as this will release more flavor.

When I make beef broth, I save a small amount in the refrigerator, where it can be safely kept for 5 to 6 days, and I freeze the rest.

Making beef broth takes a fair bit of roasting and cooking time, so you might want to use a Crock-Pot (slow cooker) and cook it over-night.

4 to 5 pounds beef shank or soup
  bones or a mixture including
  veal bones
1½ gallons cold water
1 (16-ounce) can low-sodium whole
  peeled plum tomatoes, with their
  juice
2 large ripe tomatoes, quartered
2 large yellow onions, unpeeled and
  quartered
3 large celery stalks with their leaves

3 large carrots, peeled
4 large bay leaves
1 teaspoon whole cloves
1 tablespoon whole black
  peppercorns
5 garlic cloves, unpeeled
6 large sprigs of fresh parsley
1 tablespoon dried rosemary,
  crumbled
Salt and coarsely ground black
  pepper, optional

Preheat the oven to 350°F.

Place the bones in a shallow baking pan and roast them for about

1 hour. Turn up the oven to 450°F and roast the bones for another 25 to 30 minutes.

Place the browned bones in a large, heavy pot. Deglaze the baking pan with ¼ to ½ cup water. (To deglaze a pan, place it on top of the burner or burners, add liquid — in this case, water — and while heating, scrape all of the particles from the surface with a metal spatula. The tidbits that are stuck to the pan are essential to the flavor of the broth and, coincidentally, the deglazing process makes the pan very easy to clean.)

Pour the liquid from the pan into the pot with the browned bones. Add all of the remaining ingredients. Simmer, uncovered, for about 4 hours, adding water when necessary to maintain the volume.

Remove the bones and vegetables and discard. Strain the broth through a fine-meshed strainer into a container, cool to room temperature, and refrigerate for several hours. Skim the congealed fat from the surface of the broth. Taste and correct the seasoning and add salt and pepper, if desired. Refrigerate or freeze for later use.

YIELD: 1 gallon (16 cups) SERVING SIZE: ½ cup if used as a soup

Calories	Protein	Carbohydrates	Fat	Sodium
9	0 g	2 g	0 g	18 mg

Exchange: Free

Simple Noodle Soup

This is actually one of the easiest soups in the world to make and one that will become a real family favorite. If you keep fresh chicken broth on hand or in the freezer, the soup will be ready in about 30 minutes at the most. You may use Vegetable Broth (page 128), Garlic Broth (page 132), Beef Broth (page 135), or low-fat, low-sodium canned broth if you prefer.

7 cups Chicken Broth (page 133)
   or low-fat, low-sodium canned
   broth
1 tablespoon low-fat margarine,
   optional
1 teaspoon paprika
Pinch of cayenne pepper
1 teaspoon granulated garlic or
   garlic powder

1 teaspoon salt
½ teaspoon ground white pepper
1-inch-diameter handful of dried
   fettuccine (2 to 3 ounces)
1 tablespoon fresh lime or lemon
   juice
1 tablespoon minced fresh
   parsley

In a 3- to 4-quart heavy-bottomed pot, heat the broth until it simmers.

Stir in the margarine, if desired, paprika, cayenne pepper, granulated garlic, salt, and white pepper.

Raise the heat and bring the broth to a low boil. Break the fettuccine to whatever length you prefer and add it to the broth. Lower the heat and simmer, uncovered, for 15 to 20 minutes. At this point the fettuccine should be tender.

Stir in the lime juice, ladle into bowls, sprinkle the parsley over the soup, and serve.

YIELD: 8 cups   SERVING SIZE: ½ cup

Calories	Protein	Carbohydrates	Fat	Sodium
16	0 g	3 g	0 g	136 mg

Exchange: Free

Spinach Soup

Like many of our other soup selections, this is a good winter soup. Of course, it is just as wonderful during the summer months, but since spinach is as good if not better in the winter, it is an all-year-round inexpensive soup.

Our version is light and refreshing and works perfectly with a heavier dish such as a soybean casserole or roasted chicken.

2 quarts Chicken Broth (page 133), Vegetable Broth (page 128), Garlic Broth (page 132), or low-fat, low-sodium canned broth

2 large bunches of spinach, thoroughly washed, stemmed, and drained

2 large red potatoes, peeled and cut into ½-inch dice

1 cup sliced green onions or scallions

1 teaspoon salt substitute

2 teaspoons ground white pepper

1 teaspoon granulated garlic or garlic powder

½ teaspoon ground nutmeg

½ teaspoon paprika

4 tablespoons sour cream substitute

3 tablespoons fresh lime or lemon juice

2 tablespoons minced fresh parsley or chives for garnish, optional

In a large, heavy pot over medium heat, bring the broth to a simmer.

Add the spinach, potatoes, and ½ cup of the green onions. Season with the salt substitute, white pepper, and granulated garlic and simmer over very low heat, uncovered, for about 45 minutes. Stir periodically.

Add the remaining ½ cup green onions, the nutmeg, and paprika and stir.

In a small bowl, whisk together the sour cream substitute and lime juice. Add 1 to 1½ cups of the hot soup stock to the sour cream mixture and whisk together. Take the resulting mixture and whisk it back into the soup.

Simmer for about another 45 minutes, taste and correct the seasoning, and add more lime juice if a sharper taste is desired. If you wish, serve garnished with the parsley or chives.

YIELD: 3 to 3½ quarts   SERVING SIZE: ⅔ cup

Calories	Protein	Carbohydrates	Fat	Sodium
23	1 g	4 g	0 g	13 mg

Exchange: 1 vegetable

Winter Green Soup

Most of the vegetables for this soup are seasonal winter vegetables and all of them are green. It is delicious and quite easy to put together. When served with crusty bread and a big salad, it makes a delicious lunch.

1 large yellow onion, halved lengthwise and thinly sliced

2 large celery stalks, thinly sliced

3 large garlic cloves, finely minced

1 teaspoon extra-virgin olive oil

6 cups Vegetable Broth (page 128) or low-fat, low-sodium canned broth

3/4 cup green split peas, thoroughly rinsed and drained

2 small bay leaves

4 cups zucchini, cut into 1/2-inch pieces

2 cups broccoli, cut into fairly small pieces (use only a little of the stems)

1/2 teaspoon dried basil

1/2 teaspoon ground white pepper

1/2 teaspoon salt substitute

1 large bunch of spinach, thoroughly washed, stemmed, drained, and sliced into 3-inch pieces

3 tablespoons stemmed and coarsely chopped fresh parsley

1/4 teaspoon ground nutmeg

1/4 cup thinly sliced green onions or scallions (green parts only) for garnish

In a large, heavy pot over medium heat, sauté the yellow onion, celery, and garlic in the oil until the onion is soft. Add 4 cups of the broth, the split peas, and bay leaves. Bring to a boil, lower the heat, then cover and simmer for about 45 minutes.

Add the zucchini and broccoli, the remaining broth, the basil, white pepper, and salt substitute. Cook for about 8 minutes more.

Remove the bay leaves and discard them.

Puree the soup in a blender and return it to the pot. Stir in the spinach, parsley, and nutmeg. Simmer the soup for about 5 minutes more, making sure that it is thoroughly heated.

Serve and garnish with the green onions.

YIELD: 8 cups   SERVING SIZE: ⅔ cup

Calories	*Protein*	*Carbohydrates*	*Fat*	*Sodium*
64	4.4 g	12 g	0.74 g	19 mg

Exchange: 1 starch

Beet-Top Borscht

This soup recipe uses whole fresh beets. If you are unable to find beets with their tops intact, you may substitute sliced spinach leaves, arugula, or sliced curly endive. You will want to add some sort of green leafy vegetable for the taste as well as for the color contrast it provides.

Serve this soup either hot or cold. A spoonful of plain nonfat yogurt mixed with a dash of paprika and a bit of dried dill is a delicious addition.

8 medium beets with their
   tops
1 medium russet or Yukon Gold
   potato, peeled and diced
1 large yellow onion, diced
2 tablespoons minced garlic
1 tablespoon dried dill,
   crumbled
½ teaspoon salt, optional
2 teaspoons coarsely ground black
   pepper
2 teaspoons brown sugar
   substitute

2 quarts Chicken Broth (page 133),
   Garlic Broth (page 132),
   Vegetable Broth (page 128), or
   low-fat, low-sodium canned broth
2 teaspoons canola oil
2 teaspoons whole wheat flour
Juice of 1 lime or lemon
¼ cup plain nonfat yogurt for
   topping, optional
¼ teaspoon paprika for topping,
   optional
¼ teaspoon dried dill for topping,
   optional

Scrub the beets and wash the beet tops. Chop the beet tops and set them aside. Grate the beets with a hand grater or with a food processor grater blade.

To a large soup pot, add the beets, potato, onion, garlic, dill, salt, pepper, and brown sugar substitute. Pour in the broth. Bring the mixture to a low boil over medium heat and then simmer, uncovered, until the vegetables are tender and well cooked, about 1 hour.

Meanwhile, mix the oil and flour in a small (1-quart) saucepan and cook this "roux" over low heat for about 1 minute.

Take 1 cup of the soup mixture and slowly, whisking all the while, add the soup to the roux. Stirring constantly, cook this sauce over low heat until it thickens. Return the sauce to the soup pot.

Stir in the lime juice and taste and correct the seasoning.

Add the chopped beet tops, stir, and cook the soup for 5 to 6 minutes more.

If desired, combine the yogurt, paprika, and dill and put a tablespoonful of this mixture on top of each serving.

YIELD: 3 quarts

SERVING SIZE: ⅔ cup plus 1 tablespoon yogurt mixture for topping

Calories	Protein	Carbohydrates	Fat	Sodium
21	1 g	4 g	1 g	14 mg

Exchange: 1 vegetable

Chilled Blender Borscht

Quick and easy, this is a good opener for any dinner, and leftovers make a handy snack. It will hold in the refrigerator for 2 to 3 days. You do need to chill the soup before serving.

3 green onions or scallions, white root tips trimmed off and cut into 4 pieces each

1 large cucumber, peeled, seeded, and cut into chunks

1 (16-ounce) can sliced beets, chilled in their liquid

½ cup Chicken Broth (page 133), Garlic Broth (page 132), Vegetable Broth (page 128), or low-fat, low-sodium canned broth

1 cup beet juice or prepared borscht (available in jars at most supermarkets)

1 heaping teaspoon white or red horseradish (white is spicy, red is mild)

1 tablespoon red wine vinegar

Salt and ground white pepper to taste

½ cup plain nonfat yogurt for topping, optional

2 tablespoons fresh dill, or ½ teaspoon dried, crumbled, for topping, optional

Splash of fresh lime or lemon juice for topping, optional

Put the green onions, cucumber, beets with their liquid, and broth in a blender and process for about 5 seconds. Add the beet juice, horseradish, vinegar, and salt and white pepper. Process the soup until the ingredients are pretty well mixed, but do leave the soup with some texture. Taste and correct the seasoning. Chill.

If desired, combine the yogurt, dill, and lime juice and put a tablespoonful of this mixture on top of each serving.

YIELD: 5 cups

SERVING SIZE: ½ cup plus 1 tablespoon yogurt mixture for topping

Calories	Protein	Carbohydrates	Fat	Sodium
26	1 g	5 g	0 g	96 mg

Exchange: 1 vegetable

Onion Soup

This is not the traditional French onion soup topped with melted Gruyère. But it *is* served with bread and Parmesan cheese and is quite light and delicious. It is also easy to make.

To prepare and serve this soup with croutons (slices of toasted French bread), you will need either a large ovenproof casserole or individual ovenproof casseroles. Plain Pyrex bowls work beautifully.

1 teaspoon canola oil

4 large yellow or white onions, halved lengthwise and thinly sliced

2 cups Chicken Broth (page 133), Garlic Broth (page 132), Vegetable Broth (page 128), or low-fat, low-sodium canned broth

2 cups Beef Broth (page 135) or low-fat, low-sodium canned broth

2 cups cold water

2 teaspoons fresh lime or lemon juice

1 tablespoon dry sherry

2 large bay leaves

¼ teaspoon dried thyme, crumbled

½ teaspoon dried marjoram, crumbled

Salt substitute and coarsely ground black pepper to taste

1 teaspoon ground white pepper

1 teaspoon granulated garlic or garlic powder

10 (1-ounce) slices French bread, toasted, for croutons, optional

1 tablespoon finely grated low-fat Parmesan cheese for each slice of bread, optional

In a large, heavy-bottomed ovenproof Dutch oven or a skillet with high sides, heat the oil and when it is hot, toss in the onions and sauté gently until they are very tender and golden. Pour the broths, water, lime juice, and sherry over the onions. Add the bay leaves, thyme, and marjoram. Season with the salt substitute, black and white pepper, and granulated garlic, and slowly simmer, uncovered, for 30 to 45 minutes. The soup is ready at this point if you choose not to serve with croutons.

Preheat the oven to 375°F.

Just before serving, pour the hot soup into either a large ovenproof casserole or individual ovenproof bowls. Top the large casserole with all the bread or the individual bowls with 1 slice each. Sprinkle the Parmesan cheese over the bread. Using the lower shelf of the oven, bake the soup for about 10 minutes and then serve immediately.

YIELD: **10 servings**   SERVING SIZE: ⅔ cup

Without the bread and Parmesan cheese:

Calories	*Protein*	*Carbohydrates*	*Fat*	*Sodium*
34.71	0.82 g	7.05 g	0.58 g	8.86 mg

Exchange: 1 starch

With the bread and Parmesan cheese:

Calories	*Protein*	*Carbohydrates*	*Fat*	*Sodium*
132.71	5.92 g	22.25 g	2.18 g	261.86 mg

Exchange: 1¼ starches; ½ fat

Minestrone

This soup can serve as an entrée when accompanied by a salad.

2 teaspoons extra-virgin olive oil

2 medium potatoes, peeled and cut into large cubes

3 medium carrots, peeled and sliced into ¼-inch pieces

1 medium yellow or white onion, halved lengthwise and thinly sliced

2 quarts Chicken Broth (page 133), Garlic Broth (page 132), Vegetable Broth (page 128), or low-fat, low-sodium canned broth

2 teaspoons dried basil, crumbled

½ teaspoon dried oregano, crumbled

2 teaspoons minced fresh parsley, or 1 teaspoon dried, crumbled

3 large garlic cloves, minced

5 to 6 large ripe tomatoes, peeled, or 1 (29-ounce) can low-sodium whole peeled tomatoes, drained, cut into large chunks

2 medium zucchini, cut into ½-inch slices

1 cup fresh or frozen cut green beans

¼ cup fresh or frozen corn kernels

⅓ cup cooked kidney beans or lentils

1-inch-diameter handful of spaghetti, broken into pieces (about ¼ cup)

Salt substitute to taste

Coarsely ground black pepper to taste

Several teaspoons grated Parmesan cheese for serving, optional

Heat the oil in a large soup pot and add the potatoes, carrots, and onion. Sauté the vegetables for a few minutes (until the onion is soft) and then add the broth, basil, oregano, parsley, and garlic.

Bring the soup to a low boil, lower the heat, and simmer, uncovered, for 10 to 15 minutes. Add half of the tomatoes, the zucchini, green beans, corn, and kidney beans. Simmer for about 15 minutes, and then add the spaghetti, the remaining tomatoes, and the salt substitute and pepper. Cook for another 13 to 15 minutes.

At this point the spaghetti should be al dente. Serve immediately, garnished with sprinkles of the Parmesan, if desired.

YIELD: 3 quarts   SERVING SIZE: ⅔ cup

Calories	Protein	Carbohydrates	Fat	Sodium
76	1.87 g	11.5 g	2.77 g	10 mg

Exchange: 1 starch

Carrot and Sweet Potato Soup

This family-style soup from China is particularly rich in vitamin A. The ginger and garlic give it its distinctive flavor.

It is also a good winter soup in that it does not rely on expensive, out-of-season vegetables.

6 cups Chicken Broth (page 133), Garlic Broth (page 132), Vegetable Broth (page 128), or low-fat, low-sodium canned broth

1½-inch piece fresh ginger, peeled and cut into thin slices

4 green onions, thinly sliced (use the white tips and part of the green, saving the rest of the green parts for garnish)

3 garlic cloves, thinly sliced

2½ tablespoons reduced- or low-sodium soy sauce

2 tablespoons dry sherry or sake

½ teaspoon ground white pepper

4 large carrots, peeled and cut into 1½-inch chunks

1 large sweet potato, peeled and cut into 1-inch-square chunks

1 medium to large russet or Yukon Gold potato, peeled and cut into 1-inch-square chunks

1 serrano chili, split, seeded, and finely minced

In a large (5- to 6-quart) soup pot, combine the broth, ginger, green onions, garlic, soy sauce, sherry, and white pepper and bring to a boil over medium-high heat.

Add the carrots, cover, and simmer for about 12 minutes. Add the sweet potato, russet potato, and the chili. Cover and simmer for about

40 minutes more, at which point the vegetables should be very tender when pierced with a fork.

Serve and garnish with the reserved green onions.

YIELD: 6 servings   SERVING SIZE: ⅔ cup

Calories	Protein	Carbohydrates	Fat	Sodium
69	1.50 g	14.5 g	0 g	252.50 mg

Exchange: 1 starch

Spicy Corn-and-Tortilla Soup

This soup is simple to make and very flavorful. Spicy and hearty, it works well with a tossed salad for lunch or as a first course for dinner. The soup freezes nicely, so I keep some on hand for those times when I need to put something together quickly. If you like a less spicy soup, reduce the number of chilies.

6 low-sodium corn tortillas

1 large yellow onion, halved lengthwise and thinly sliced

4 cups Chicken Broth (page 133), Garlic Broth (page 132), Vegetable Broth (page 128), or low-fat, low-sodium canned broth

1 (46-ounce) can low-sodium tomato juice

1½ cups fresh or frozen corn kernels

1 (14½-ounce) can low-sodium whole peeled plum tomatoes, coarsely chopped, with their juice

5 serrano chilies, or 3 jalapeño peppers

3 tablespoons minced garlic

1 tablespoon coarsely ground black pepper

1 tablespoon chili powder, or to taste

1 teaspoon dried oregano, crumbled

½ teaspoon ground cumin

Salt substitute to taste, optional

Pico de Gallo Salsa (page 170) for garnish, optional

2 ounces reduced-fat grated Monterey Jack cheese for garnish, optional

Coarsely chop the corn tortillas and put them with the onion and the broth into a large, heavy pot. Bring the mixture to a boil, lower the heat, and add the tomato juice, corn, and tomatoes. Stir.

If using serrano chilies, halve 3 of them lengthwise, remove the seeds, and thinly slice. If adding jalapeño peppers, use only 2, halved lengthwise, seeded, and thinly sliced. Add to the broth mixture. Reserve the remaining whole chilies for garnish.

Stir the broth mixture and add the garlic, pepper, chili powder, oregano, cumin, and salt substitute, if desired.

Simmer, partially covered, for about 1½ hours. If necessary, add more broth to maintain the volume of the soup. If you wish, serve garnished with the Pico de Gallo Salsa or the grated cheese and the remaining serrano chilies, seeded and minced.

YIELD: 8 cups   SERVING SIZE: ⅔ cup

Using Pico de Gallo garnish:

Calories	Protein	Carbohydrates	Fat	Sodium
92.34	3.2 g	17.65 g	0.44 g	72.94 mg

Using cheese and chili garnish:

Calories	Protein	Carbohydrates	Fat	Sodium
121.34	5.65 g	19.85 g	1.70 g	121.14 mg

Exchange: 1½ vegetables; ½ bread; add ½ lean meat if using cheese garnish

Lime-Tarragon French Fish Soup (Pot-au-Feu)

For this fish soup, you will want a firm-fleshed white fish, such as flounder, snapper, rockfish, black drum, redfish, or orange roughy. I use tarragon in this soup as the predominant herb and flavor; however, you may use basil, rosemary, dill, marjoram, or whatever your favorite herb might be. Unlike many fish soups, this soup is light and herbal in taste and very colorful in its presentation.

6 cups Chicken Broth (page 133), Garlic Broth (page 132), Vegetable Broth (page 128), or low-fat, low-sodium canned broth

1 cup dry white wine

2 tablespoons fresh tarragon, finely chopped, or 1 teaspoon dried (see headnote)

½ teaspoon ground white pepper

½ teaspoon salt

8 tiny new potatoes (about 1 pound), thoroughly scrubbed

1 small yellow onion, halved lengthwise and each half quartered

8 very small, slender carrots, peeled

4 small leeks, root ends trimmed, halved lengthwise, and thoroughly soaked and rinsed (see Note)

1 pound skinned and boned white, firm-fleshed fish, cut into 4 (4-ounce) pieces

3 tablespoons fresh lime or lemon juice

In a large (6-quart) pot, combine the broth, wine, tarragon, white pepper, and salt and bring to a boil over medium heat. Add the potatoes, onion, and carrots and return to a boil. Lower the heat, cover, and simmer for 10 to 12 minutes.

Add the leeks to the pot. Cover and simmer until the leeks are tender when tested with a knife. This should take about 10 to 12 minutes. Remove the leeks from the soup and set aside.

Add the fish and lime juice to the soup, cover, and simmer until the fish is firm and whitish in color and the vegetables are tender.

To serve, place the leeks in wide soup bowls, then add the fish, vegetables, and broth.

NOTE: When cooking with leeks, it is extremely important to soak and rinse them thoroughly, as they can be very dirty. For this recipe, discard most of the green tops before washing so that the trimmed leeks are about 6 inches long. This will make cleaning a little easier.

YIELD: 4 servings

SERVING SIZE: 1 cup broth plus 1 portion (3 ounces) fish, 2 carrots, 2 potatoes, and 1 leek

Calories	Protein	Carbohydrates	Fat	Sodium
257	20 g	32 g	1 g	145 mg

Exchange: 3 lean meats; 1 bread; 2 vegetables

Northwest Cioppino

Cioppino is a mixed seafood stew from the West Coast. This thick, hearty soup-stew serves easily as an entrée and is delicious accompanied by a good bread and a crisp tossed green salad. For the fish in the cioppino, I use snapper, perch, flounder, or any other white, firm-fleshed fish or any nonoily firm-fleshed fish.

Nonstick cooking spray for sautéing

2 cups thinly sliced yellow onions

2 tablespoons finely minced garlic

1½ (16-ounce) cans low-sodium whole peeled plum tomatoes, coarsely chopped, with their juice

1 (8-ounce) can low-sodium tomato sauce

½ cup cold water

½ cup dry white wine

¼ cup coarsely chopped fresh parsley

1 teaspoon salt substitute

1½ teaspoons dried basil, crumbled

½ teaspoon dried oregano, crumbled

½ teaspoon ground white pepper

½ pound fresh or frozen scallops (if the scallops are unusually large, cut them in half; if frozen, thaw them)

½ pound skinned and boned firm-fleshed fish, cut into 1-inch chunks

½ cup diced red bell pepper

1 cup cooked, peeled, and deveined medium shrimp (36 to 42 shrimp per pound)

2 teaspoons fresh lime or lemon juice

¼ cup chopped fresh cilantro leaves

Spray a large, heavy pot with the nonstick cooking spray and heat over medium heat. Toss in the onions and garlic and sauté until the onions are tender but not browned.

Add the tomatoes, tomato sauce, water, wine, parsley, salt substitute, basil, oregano, and white pepper. Cover and gently simmer for about 30 minutes.

Add the scallops and the fish, cover, and simmer for about 15 minutes, or until the fish chunks flake with a fork.

Add the bell pepper, shrimp, and lime juice and simmer for 5 minutes more, or until the shrimp are heated. Stir in the cilantro, ladle into bowls, and serve.

YIELD: 3½ quarts   SERVING SIZE: 1¼ cups

Calories	Protein	Carbohydrates	Fat	Sodium
103	13 g	7 g	1.5 g	200 mg

Exchange: 2 lean meats; 1 vegetable

Mulligatawny Soup (Stew)

Mulligatawny soup was brought to Britain from India in the nineteenth century. The name comes from a Tamil word meaning "hot" or "pepper water." Although this recipe is certainly less spicy than the traditional version, it is still full of flavor and serves as a perfect counterpoint when served over a bland starch such as rice or plain semolina noodles.

This soup may be made a day ahead, covered, refrigerated, and served the next.

1½ teaspoons canola oil

1 pound boneless, skinless chicken parts (breasts, thighs, legs), trimmed of excess fat

2 medium yellow onions, finely diced

3 celery stalks, thinly sliced

1 large carrot, peeled and finely diced

2½ tablespoons good-quality curry powder

½ teaspoon ground tumeric

2 tablespoons finely minced garlic

1 quart Chicken Broth (page 133), Garlic Broth (page 132), Vegetable Broth (page 128), or low-fat, low-sodium canned broth

2½ cups unsweetened natural apple juice

¾ cup dried lentils

Salt substitute to taste

Cayenne pepper to taste (for a milder, less-fiery taste, use black pepper instead)

3 medium potatoes, peeled and chopped into small dice

1½ teaspoons dried dill, crumbled

2 tablespoons fresh lime or lemon juice

½ cup plain nonfat yogurt

½ small tart apple, peeled and diced

2 tablespoons chopped fresh cilantro leaves

1 to 1½ cups cooked rice or noodles

Heat the oil in a large, heavy-bottomed soup pot over medium heat and add the chicken, onions, celery, and carrot. Sprinkle with the curry powder and turmeric, cover, lower the heat, and cook, stirring occasionally, for about 15 minutes.

Add the garlic, broth, apple juice, lentils, salt substitute, and cayenne pepper. Simmer, uncovered, over low heat, for about 20 minutes.

Add the potatoes, dill, and lime juice, cover, and simmer for about 25 minutes more.

Stir the soup, making sure the vegetables and chicken are thoroughly dispersed.

In a small bowl, combine the yogurt, apple, and cilantro. Serve the soup over ¼ cup of rice or noodles and top with 1 heaping tablespoon of the yogurt mixture.

YIELD: 6 servings

SERVING SIZE: ⅔ cup soup over ¼ cup rice or noodles

Calories	Protein	Carbohydrates	Fat	Sodium
367	26 g	50 g	7.67 g	100 mg

Exchange: 2 starches; 1 fruit; 3 lean meats

Sauces, Salsas, Chutneys, and Relishes

Ancho Chili Sauce

Tomatillo Sauce (*Salsa Verdes*)

Cranberry Sauce

Cranberry Salsa

Pico de Gallo Salsa

Marinara Sauce

Jiffy Marinara Sauce

Spicy Pineapple Chutney

Cranberry Chutney

Fresh Cranberry, Tangerine, and Lime Relish

Pear Relish

Pickled Bell Peppers

Ancho Chili Sauce

The ancho is a dried poblano pepper. It is aromatic with a sweet and very rich flavor. It is the most popular dried chili in Mexico and is starting to become very popular in the United States. It can be stored in a Ziploc bag, unrefrigerated, in a fairly cool, dry place for months.

In this recipe, I also use sun-dried tomatoes. I prefer to get the dehydrated ones at the market and rehydrate them myself. I don't buy the ones in jars, which are packed in olive oil, because not only do they have all that extra fat from the oil, they are much more expensive.

The sauce is made in two stages. First, you make the puree, which may be stored in the refrigerator for a month or so or may be frozen for future use. Then you use the puree to make the sauce, which takes about 40 minutes. You can make the puree one day and make the sauce another, or you can do them the same day. Ancho sauce is delicious with roasted chicken, Baked Chiles Rellenos (page 302), enchiladas, and even fish. It also works well as a glaze when you are grilling or broiling meats or fish.

6 to 7 ancho chilies, stemmed and
    seeded
4 sun-dried tomatoes, rehydrated
    (see Note)
3 tablespoons fresh lime or lemon juice
2 tablespoons apple cider vinegar
1 tablespoon honey
1 quart Chicken Broth (page 133),
    Garlic Broth (page 132),
    Vegetable Broth (page 128), or
    low-fat, low-sodium canned broth

2 cups water
Nonstick cooking spray for
    sautéing
1 small yellow onion, finely diced
2 tablespoons finely minced garlic
2 teaspoons ground cumin
2 teaspoons dried oregano, crumbled
1 large bay leaf
2 tablespoons cornstarch mixed
    with 3 tablespoons cold water,
    optional

Place the chilies, sun-dried tomatoes, 2 tablespoons of the lime juice, the vinegar, honey, 1 cup of the broth, and the water in a medium saucepan, bring to a boil, and then simmer, uncovered, until the chilies have softened (about 25 minutes). If necessary, add a bit more broth to the broth mixture as it simmers to maintain the volume.

When the chilies are properly softened, put the entire mixture into a blender or food processor and thoroughly puree. Set the puree aside.

Heat a medium, heavy saucepan, coat it with the nonstick cooking spray, and when it is hot, add the onion and sauté until the onion is soft. Add the remainder of the broth, bring it to a slow boil, and whisk in about ½ cup of the puree. Add the garlic, cumin, oregano, bay leaf, and the remaining 1 tablespoon of lime juice. Let the mixture cook, uncovered, for about 20 minutes and taste it. If it does not taste strong enough, add 3 to 4 more tablespoons of the puree and cook an additional 15 minutes.

Normally the sauce is thick enough on its own, but if you have the taste you want and not the consistency, stir the cornstarch mixture and then whisk the mixture into the sauce. Cook for 3 to 4 minutes, remove the bay leaf, and serve.

N O T E : To rehydrate sun-dried tomatoes, boil them in water for about 5 minutes until soft, drain thoroughly, and use.

Y I E L D : 3 cups puree (½ cup   S E R V I N G S I Z E : 3 to 4 tablespoons
puree yields 3 cups sauce)

Calories	Protein	Carbohydrates	Fat	Sodium
17	0 g	4 g	0 g	0 mg

Exchange: Free

VARIATIONS

Enchilada Sauce: Substitute 8 to 10 red (mild, medium, or hot) New Mexico or California chilies for the ancho chilies.

Ancho Chili Glaze: Make the puree. In a small saucepan, thin ½ cup of the puree with 1 cup of the broth and bring to a boil. Meanwhile, mix together 1 tablespoon cornstarch with 2 tablespoons cold water in a small soup bowl. Pour this mixture into the boiling sauce, reduce the heat, and simmer, uncovered, for about 5 minutes, until the desired consistency is reached.

I use the glaze to grill or broil chicken, fish, or beef. Coat the surface of the meat with the glaze and cook as usual, basting periodically during the process.

Tomatillo Sauce (Salsa Verdes)

Tomatillos, also known as jamberries, are the fruit of a plant in the tomato family and are grown in Central and South America as well as parts of the southern United States. The edible berry, encased in a loose-fitting parchmentlike husk, should be bright green in color. The husk is removed and then the tomatillo can be broiled, baked, or sautéed. They can be eaten raw but are much more flavorful when cooked. The easiest way to remove the husk is to put the fruit in a colander in the sink and peel the husk off as you are washing it prior to cooking.

Tomatillo sauce is delicious with traditional southwestern cuisine, such as enchiladas, Baked Chiles Rellenos (page 302), or nachos, and is just as delicious when served with roasted chicken, broiled or grilled fish, grilled meats, or eggs. It can also be used as a dip with chips. Tomatillo sauce will keep for 4 to 5 days easily in the refrigerator and may also be frozen for future use.

1½ pounds firm, ripe tomatillos
5 or 6 green onions or scallions
1 large bunch of cilantro, leaves picked and stems discarded
4 to 5 small serrano chilies, or 2 medium jalapeño peppers
¼ cup finely minced garlic
2 to 3 tablespoons fresh lime or lemon juice, or to taste

½ teaspoon salt substitute
2 teaspoons granulated sugar substitute, or to taste
1 cup Chicken Broth (page 133), Garlic Broth (page 132), Vegetable Broth (page 128), or low-fat, low-sodium canned broth

Put the tomatillos in a colander in the sink and with the water running, remove the husks from the tomatillos. Place the tomatillos in a shallow broilerproof pan and broil until nicely browned. Remove the pan from the broiler and turn the tomatillos over, return the pan to the broiler, and repeat the process until the tomatillos are browned all over.

Put the tomatillos, with the pan juices, into a food processor with a steel blade. Add the green onions, cilantro, chilies, garlic, lime juice, salt substitute, and sugar substitute. Process until the mixture is thoroughly combined. With the machine running, gradually add the broth until the mixture is completely blended. Taste and add more lime juice if necessary.

The tomatillo sauce may be served at room temperature or may be heated. However, if the sauce is heated for longer than a few minutes, it will lose some of its vibrant color.

YIELD: 1 quart   SERVING SIZE: ¼ cup

Calories	Protein	Carbohydrates	Fat	Sodium
13	0 g	3 g	0 g	20 mg

Exchange: Free

Cranberry Sauce

Cranberry sauce is so simple to make that you will find yourself using it to complement more than just the Thanksgiving turkey. It is delicious with all poultry, game, beans, rice, and couscous. You might want to buy extra cranberries when they are available in November and December and freeze them for later use. The frozen berries need not be thawed before using.

This sauce requires very little cooking time but does take several hours to chill. It will keep in the refrigerator for 2 to 3 weeks.

3 cups (12 ounces) fresh or
  frozen cranberries (see
  headnote)
1 cup water

½ cup plus 1 tablespoon granulated
  sugar substitute
1½ to 2 tablespoons fresh lime or
  lemon juice

Thoroughly rinse and drain the cranberries.

Over high heat, bring the water to a rolling boil in a large (10- or 12-inch) skillet. Add the cranberries, sugar substitute, and lime juice.

Lower the heat to medium and simmer, uncovered, until the skins of the cranberries start to pop (about 8 minutes).

Skim any white foam from the sauce. Pour the cranberry sauce into a dish to cool. When the mixture is cool, cover, refrigerate for at least 2 hours, and serve.

YIELD: 2½ cups   SERVING SIZE: 3 to 4
                                              tablespoons

Calories	Protein	Carbohydrates	Fat	Sodium
14	0 g	4 g	0 g	0 mg

Exchange: Free

Cranberry Salsa

This salsa is delicious with grilled fish or chicken as well as with roasted turkey. It also complements beans, rice, and couscous. It may be kept in the refrigerator for 2 to 3 weeks.

1¾ cups Cranberry Sauce (page 167), or 1 (14-ounce) can sugar-free whole cranberry sauce
1 small red onion, finely chopped

2 jalapeño peppers, seeded and finely chopped
Grated zest and juice of 1 large lime or lemon

Thoroughly combine all of the ingredients and chill. Serve.

YIELD: 2 cups

SERVING SIZE: 3 to 4 tablespoons

Calories	Protein	Carbohydrates	Fat	Sodium
12	0 g	3 g	0 g	0 mg

Exchange: Free

Pico de Gallo Salsa

Salsas have been an important element in Mexican and southwestern cuisine for years, and now they have replaced catsup as the most popular condiment in the United States. A condiment is simply a flavor enhancer, and salsa certainly is that. There are many salsas, but my favorite is this variation of pico de gallo. It is spicy and full of vegetables and is a healthy enhancer of food. It is delicious served with enchiladas, Baked Chiles Rellenos (page 302), tacos, chicken, fish, or beef. It works quite well with eggs and with chips as a dip. It is quickly assembled and can be kept in the refrigerator for several weeks.

6 ripe medium plum tomatoes, or 3 large ripe Beefsteak tomatoes, cut into medium dice

1 small red onion, finely diced

4 green onions or scallions, thinly sliced

4 small serrano chilies, or 2 medium jalapeño peppers, seeded and minced (for spicier salsa, leave in the seeds)

3 tablespoons minced garlic

1 large bunch of cilantro, leaves picked and stems discarded

½ teaspoon salt

3 to 4 tablespoons fresh lime juice (add 1 to 2 teaspoons more for a sharper taste)

In a glass or acid-resistant bowl, gently combine the tomatoes, red and green onions, chilies, garlic, cilantro, salt, and lime juice.

Let the salsa sit for 20 to 30 minutes before serving. Store the unused portion in the refrigerator."

YIELD: 1 quart   SERVING SIZE: ¼ cup

Calories	Protein	Carbohydrates	Fat	Sodium
10	0 g	2 g	0 g	22 mg

Exchange: Free

Marinara Sauce

I make this marinara sauce in large quantities when I have both the time and the room on the stove to do it. The sauce, which I store in containers in the freezer, has been part of many a meal at my house and saved my time as well. It works well with all sorts of pasta dishes as well as with more complicated meals for my family and friends. With this sauce on hand, lasagne, manicotti, stuffed calzone, and pizza are quick and easy. If you don't have the time to make this sauce, the recipe for Jiffy Marinara Sauce (page 173) will enable you to make the same dishes with ease. It does not, however, taste the same as a sauce that you cook for a longer period of time.

2 (29-ounce) cans low-sodium
  whole peeled plum tomatoes,
  coarsely chopped, with their juice;
  or 16 large ripe plum tomatoes,
  peeled and coarsely chopped
1 cup dry red wine
2 (29-ounce) cans low-sodium
  tomato sauce
1 quart Chicken Broth (page 133),
  Garlic Broth (page 132), or low-
  fat, low-sodium canned broth
3 medium yellow onions, halved
  lengthwise and thinly sliced
4 (3-ounce) packages frozen
  artichoke hearts, thawed
3 large red bell peppers (yellow or
  green may be substituted),
  stemmed, seeded, and cut into
  medium dice

3 cups (about 1 pound) sliced brown
  mushrooms
5 celery stalks, thinly sliced
¼ cup finely minced garlic
Coarsely ground black pepper to
  taste
Salt substitute to taste, optional
2 tablespoons dried basil, crumbled,
  or ⅓ cup sliced fresh leaves
1½ tablespoons dried oregano,
  crumbled, or ½ cup fresh leaves
1½ tablespoons crushed fennel
  seeds
2 teaspoons crushed red pepper
  flakes
2 tablespoons balsamic vinegar
1 tablespoon granulated sugar
  substitute
Juice of 1 lime or lemon

Crush the tomatoes in your hands and put them in a large pot (3 gallons or more). If using canned tomatoes, add the liquid. Pour in ¾ cup of the red wine, tomato sauce, and broth. Thoroughly combine.

Heat the mixture to a low boil and add the onions, artichoke hearts, bell peppers, mushrooms, celery, and garlic. Stir to combine. Add the black pepper, salt substitute, if desired, basil, oregano, fennel seeds, red pepper flakes, balsamic vinegar, and sugar substitute.

Lower the heat, cover, and simmer for about 1½ hours, stirring periodically.

Add the remaining ¼ cup of wine and the lime juice and simmer, covered, for 1 hour more, stirring occasionally. The sauce should be done at this point. If you want more flavor, cook for about 30 minutes more. Serve hot, or cool to room temperature and refrigerate or freeze.

YIELD: 1½ gallons   SERVING SIZE: ½ cup

Calories	Protein	Carbohydrates	Fat	Sodium
36.37	1.09 g	7.37 g	0 g	21.76 mg

Exchange: 1 vegetable

Jiffy Marinara Sauce

When I don't have any sauce in the freezer or change my menu at the last minute, this is the sauce I use. It works beautifully with spaghetti, linguini, or fettuccine for a quick meal. And it works equally well when you are making lasagne or manicotti or need a sauce for pizza. The sauce will keep nicely in the refrigerator for 4 to 5 days and can also be frozen for future use.

Nonstick cooking spray for sautéing

1 small yellow onion, finely diced

1½ tablespoons minced garlic

½ small red bell pepper, stemmed,
seeded, and diced

1 (35-ounce) can low-sodium whole
peeled plum tomatoes, coarsely
chopped, with their juice

2 tablespoons dry red wine

1 teaspoon crushed fennel seeds

2 tablespoons minced fresh basil, or
2 teaspoons dried, crumbled

1 teaspoon dried oregano, crumbled

1 teaspoon coarsely ground black
pepper

Heat a large (10- or 12-inch), heavy-bottomed skillet over medium heat. When the pan is hot, lightly coat it with the nonstick cooking spray and sauté the onion, garlic, and bell pepper until the onion starts to soften.

Add the tomatoes and their liquid, red wine, fennel seeds, basil, oregano, and black pepper. Cover and continue cooking over medium heat, stirring frequently, until the sauce starts to develop some flavor (about 5 minutes).

Lower the heat, remove the cover, and simmer, stirring occasionally, until the sauce thickens (about 8 minutes more) and has a nice flavor. Remove from the heat and serve.

YIELD: 1 quart

SERVING SIZE: 4 to 6
tablespoons

Calories	Protein	Carbohydrates	Fat	Sodium
29	1 g	5 g	0 g	157 mg

Exchange: 1 vegetable

Spicy Pineapple Chutney

Chutney is a sweet-and-sour condiment that originated in India in the middle of the nineteenth century. It is delicious served with curries, beans, rice, meats, poultry, or fish.

For this chutney, use fresh pineapple. If, however, fresh pineapple is too expensive or cannot easily be found, canned pineapple chunks with no salt and no sugar can be substituted, although the flavor and texture will not be the same.

This chutney will keep for 4 to 5 weeks in the refrigerator. It needs about 1½ hours cooking time and should sit for several days before you use it to allow the flavors to develop.

4 cups peeled, cored, and cubed fresh pineapple, or drained sugar-free canned chunks

¾ cup brown sugar substitute or Sucanat

2 ripe medium pears, unpeeled and cut into large dice

2 tablespoons balsamic or aged red wine vinegar

⅓ to ½ cup fresh lime or lemon juice

1 large red or green bell pepper, stemmed, seeded, and cut into medium dice

Juice of 1 orange

6 small serrano chilies, or 3 medium jalapeño peppers, seeded and finely diced

5 tablespoons finely minced garlic

1 large red onion, finely diced

½ teaspoon good-quality curry powder

½ teaspoon ground cinnamon

½ teaspoon ground allspice

¼ teaspoon ground coriander

Mix all of the ingredients in a large, heavy nonreactive saucepan and bring to a boil over high heat.

Turn down the heat to low and simmer, covered, until the taste develops. This will take 1 to 1½ hours.

When the chutney tastes good to you, remove it from the heat and pour it into a bowl and let it rest until it is completely cooled. Cover and refrigerate for several days to allow the flavors to blend.

YIELD: 6 cups   SERVING SIZE: 3 to 4 tablespoons

Calories	Protein	Carbohydrates	Fat	Sodium
27	0 g	7 g	0 g	1 mg

Exchange: ½ fruit

Cranberry Chutney

This chutney is delicious with meats, poultry, or fish, but it is also great with rice, couscous, or beans. It may be served either hot or chilled. If you want to serve it cold, allow about 1½ hours chilling time before you use it. It may be held for a month or so in the refrigerator.

1 cup dried apricots

½ cup unsweetened natural apple juice

½ cup fresh orange juice or juice made from frozen unsweetened concentrate

1 (12-ounce) package fresh or frozen whole cranberries

1 large tart apple (Granny Smith or Gala), cored and cut into medium dice

3 tablespoons minced or grated fresh ginger

2 teaspoons ground cinnamon

1 teaspoon ground cardamom

1 teaspoon ground coriander

½ teaspoon mustard seeds

2 tablespoons brown sugar substitute or Sucanat

1 tablespoon white vinegar

3 tablespoons fresh lime or lemon juice

Cut the dried apricots into small pieces with kitchen shears and set aside.

In a medium saucepan, bring the apple and orange juices to a boil over medium heat. Remove from the heat and put the chopped apricots into the hot juice mixture. Soak the apricots for about 30 minutes. This can be done ahead of time.

Add the cranberries, apple, and spices to the apricot and juice mixture, stir, and simmer over low heat, uncovered, until the cranberries pop open and are somewhat tender (about 15 minutes).

Add the brown sugar substitute, vinegar, and lime juice, stir, and simmer for about 10 minutes more.

Cranberry chutney may be served hot, at room temperature, or cold. If you wish to serve it cold, cool completely before refrigerating, cover, and chill about 1½ hours.

YIELD: 4 cups

SERVING SIZE: 3 to 4 tablespoons

Calories	Protein	Carbohydrates	Fat	Sodium
38	0 g	10 g	0 g	0 mg

Exchange: 1 fruit

Fresh Cranberry, Tangerine, and Lime Relish

This relish uses either fresh or frozen cranberries. It will keep for at least 6 weeks in the refrigerator or can be frozen.

2 medium tangerines or mandarin
   oranges, unpeeled
1 (12-ounce) package fresh or
   frozen whole cranberries

½ cup granulated sugar
   substitute
Grated zest and juice of 1 lime

Slice the unpeeled tangerines into eighths, being sure to remove the seeds. Place half of the cranberries and half of the tangerines in a food processor with a steel blade and process until smooth. Transfer the contents to a bowl. Repeat the procedure with the remaining cranberries and tangerines. Add the second batch to the bowl and stir thoroughly.

Stir in the sugar substitute, lime zest, and lime juice. Mix thoroughly. Cover and chill in the refrigerator until ready to use.

YIELD: 2½ cups

SERVING SIZE: 3 to 4 tablespoons

Calories	Protein	Carbohydrates	Fat	Sodium
14	0 g	7 g	0 g	0 mg

Exchange: Free

Pear Relish

Pear relish is best if it is held for at least 24 hours after it is made, but in a pinch it can be used after sitting for several hours. It is delicious with grilled meats, poultry, fish, beans, rice, or couscous.

For the proper texture, cut the fruit and vegetables into medium dice.

2 cups diced red bell peppers

1 teaspoon salt substitute

4 cups peeled, cored, and diced ripe
pears

2 cups diced yellow onions

1/4 cup Dijon-style mustard

1/2 cup apple cider vinegar

1/4 cup fresh lime or lemon juice

1/2 cup granulated sugar substitute

1 1/2 teaspoons celery seeds

1 teaspoon mustard seeds

1 teaspoon ground coriander

2 teaspoons ground ginger

1 teaspoon cayenne pepper

Mix together the bell peppers and salt substitute.

Combine all the ingredients in a large saucepan and gradually bring to a boil over medium heat.

Lower the heat and gently simmer, uncovered, for about 45 minutes. If necessary, skim the foam from the surface of the mixture.

Remove the pan from the heat and completely cool before storing covered in the refrigerator.

YIELD: 1 quart

SERVING SIZE: 4 to 5 tablespoons

Calories	Protein	Carbohydrates	Fat	Sodium
52	0 g	12 g	3 g	111 mg

Exchange: 1 fruit

Pickled Bell Peppers

These pickled peppers are quick and easy to make and they need only 24 hours' rest before serving. They make a really nice food gift and are a delicious accompaniment to rice, bean, meat, and fish dishes. I find it visually pleasing to use 3 different colors of bell peppers, but using only 2 colors works just fine and tastes exactly the same.

4 large bell peppers (2 green, 1 red,
   and 1 yellow)
4 cups water
½ cup apple cider vinegar
¼ cup granulated sugar substitute
1½ tablespoons pickling spice

½ to 1 teaspoon salt
¼ teaspoon ground ginger
½ teaspoon mustard seeds
1 large bay leaf
4 whole cloves
1 tablespoon minced garlic

Cut the bell peppers into 1-inch squares, saving the tops and seeds.

Heat the water, vinegar, and pepper tops and seeds in a large nonreactive pot over medium heat. When the liquid begins to come to a low boil, add all of the other ingredients except the peppers. Whisk together to make sure that everything is well mixed and then add the peppers.

Immediately turn down the heat and gently simmer the peppers, uncovered, for about 15 minutes. At this point they should be just tender. Remove the pot from the heat and let the mixture stand for another 20 minutes. Using a slotted spoon, transfer the peppers to a jar. Strain the liquid over the peppers to cover completely. Don't worry if some seeds get into the pepper mixture.

Cover the jar with waxed paper and let the jar stand unrefrigerated for about 24 hours. Serve and refrigerate the unused portion.

YIELD: 1 quart   SERVING SIZE: ¼ cup

Calories	Protein	Carbohydrates	Fat	Sodium
10	0 g	2 g	0 g	44 mg

Exchange: Free

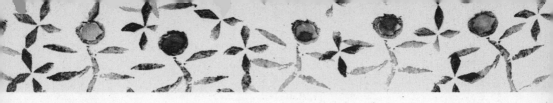

Salads

🌶

Cabbage Salad

Spicy Red Coleslaw

Curried Carrot Salad

Caraway, Cabbage, and Apple Salad

Cauliflower and Mixed Pepper Salad

Spinach, Tomato, and Red Onion Salad

Dilled Cucumber Salad

Persian Cucumber Salad

Barley, Cucumber, and Tomato Salad
with Yogurt Dressing

Mediterranean Salad

Greek Salad

Vegetable Salad with Feta Cheese

Lentil Salad

Bulgur Wheat Salad (Tabbouleh)

Tomatoes Stuffed with Vegetable Pasta Salad

Thai Tofu Salad

Southwestern Chicken Salad

Crunchy Chicken Salad

Cabbage Salad

Delicious served with Roasted Chicken Breasts (page 266). This salad requires several hours to rest in the marinade.

1¼ cups finely chopped green cabbage, Chinese cabbage, or bok choy
6 cherry tomatoes, cut into quarters, or 1 ripe medium tomato, coarsely chopped
⅔ cup finely grated peeled carrots
1 small celery stalk, finely diced
1 to 2 small serrano chilies, seeded and finely minced

1 teaspoon granulated garlic
½ teaspoon salt
1 teaspoon granulated sugar substitute
Grated zest and juice of 1 lime or lemon
½ small bunch of cilantro, leaves only (discard the stems), chopped

In a large bowl, combine the cabbage, tomatoes, carrots, celery, and chilies. In a small bowl, mix the granulated garlic, salt, sugar substitute, and lime zest and juice. Toss the vegetable mixture with the dressing, cover, and refrigerate for several hours.

Toss with the cilantro and serve.

YIELD: 6 servings   SERVING SIZE: ½ cup

Calories	Protein	Carbohydrates	Fat	Sodium
12	0 g	3 g	0 g	13 mg

Exchange: Free

Spicy Red Coleslaw

This salad is quick and easy to assemble, but it needs to be refrigerated for at least 45 minutes. It can be held in the refrigerator for up to 5 hours and remain crisp.

4 cups very finely shredded red
   cabbage
⅔ cup thinly sliced red radishes
⅔ cup peeled and shredded
   carrots
3 tablespoons finely minced fresh
   parsley
¼ cup diced red onion
¼ cup finely diced celery

1 recipe dressing (recipe follows)
Coarsely ground white pepper to
   taste
4 to 6 large crisp green-leaf lettuce
   leaves
¼ cup coarsely chopped fresh
   cilantro leaves for garnish
¼ cup thinly sliced green onions or
   scallions for garnish

In a large bowl, mix the cabbage, radishes, carrots, parsley, red onion, and celery. Toss to make sure that they are completely mixed.

Add the dressing to the coleslaw, sprinkle with the white pepper, and toss gently.

Tightly cover and refrigerate for at least 45 minutes.

When you are ready to serve, mound each serving of coleslaw on the lettuce leaves and garnish with cilantro and green onions.

Dressing

2 tablespoons fresh lime juice   –   ¼ teaspoon celery seeds
1½ tablespoons balsamic vinegar   ½ teaspoon ground cumin
1 teaspoon sugar substitute   ½ teaspoon minced garlic
1 teaspoon Dijon-style mustard   1½ tablespoons olive oil

Whisk together all of the ingredients in a small bowl, whisking in the oil last.

YIELD: 4 to 6 servings   SERVING SIZE: ¾ cup

Calories	Protein	Carbohydrates	Fat	Sodium
52	1 g	4 g	4 g	38 mg

Exchange: 1 vegetable; 1 fat

Curried Carrot Salad

2 cups peeled and grated carrots

2 tablespoons grated yellow onion

½ cup black, red, or white currants or raisins

2 teaspoons good-quality curry powder

¼ teaspoon ground cumin

Pinch of ground allspice

Pinch of cayenne pepper

Finely ground black pepper to taste

1 tablespoon canola oil

Juice of 1 lime

In a large bowl, toss the carrots with the onion and currants. In a small bowl, mix curry powder, cumin, allspice, and cayenne and black pepper with the oil and lime juice. Pour the dressing over the carrot mixture and toss. Chill and serve.

YIELD: 4 servings   SERVING SIZE: ½ cup

Calories	Protein	Carbohydrates	Fat	Sodium
108	1 g	19 g	4 g	22 mg

Exchange: 1 vegetable; 1 fruit; ½ fat

Caraway, Cabbage, and Apple Salad

You need to make the dressing for this salad ahead of time and chill it in the refrigerator for at least 1½ hours. It can be refrigerated all day or overnight.

Dressing

1 tablespoon apple cider vinegar
1½ teaspoons caraway seeds
1 teaspoon Dijon-style mustard

1 teaspoon garlic powder
¼ teaspoon salt, optional
¾ cup plain nonfat yogurt

Salad

1 large red apple (Gala or Red Delicious), cored and cut into chunks
2 teaspoons fresh lime juice
1 cup finely shredded green cabbage

1 cup finely shredded red cabbage
1 medium celery stalk, finely diced
1 tablespoon minced fresh parsley for garnish

To prepare the dressing, in a small bowl, combine the vinegar, caraway seeds, mustard, garlic powder, and salt, if desired.

In a separate bowl, whisk the yogurt until it is more liquid and then fold into the vinegar mixture. Cover and refrigerate for at least 1½ hours.

To prepare the salad, coat the apple with the lime juice. When you are ready to serve, mix the dressing with the apple, add the cabbage and celery, and toss. Garnish with the parsley and serve immediately.

YIELD: 4 servings　　　　　　　　SERVING SIZE: ½ cup

Calories	Protein	Carbohydrates	Fat	Sodium
69	3 g	14 g	0 g	80 mg

Exchange: ½ fruit; 1 vegetable

Cauliflower and Mixed Pepper Salad

This salad is not only very colorful but also delicious. I like to serve the salad in lettuce cups, for the taste as well as for the presentation. To make each cup, take apart a head of Bibb lettuce, leaf by leaf, and arrange 2 leaves to form a cup.

The salad needs to rest in the dressing for at least 1 hour before serving to allow its flavors to develop. It may be held in the refrigerator several hours before serving.

Dressing

2 tablespoons red wine vinegar
½ teaspoon salt, optional
½ teaspoon ground white pepper
2 teaspoons minced fresh
    marjoram, or ½ teaspoon dried,
    crumbled
½ teaspoon dry mustard

1 teaspoon minced garlic, or ¼
    teaspoon garlic powder
Dash of fresh lime juice
2 teaspoons canola oil
2 teaspoons extra-virgin olive
    oil

Salad

2 cups thinly sliced cauliflower
    florets
¼ cup julienned red bell pepper
¼ cup julienned yellow bell pepper
¼ cup julienned green bell pepper

¼ cup finely diced celery
12 Bibb lettuce leaves, washed,
    crisped, and formed into cups, for
    serving, optional

To make the dressing, in a small bowl, mix the vinegar and salt, if desired, and then add the white pepper, marjoram, mustard, garlic, and lime juice. Whisk the mixture thoroughly and let it rest for a few minutes. In a separate bowl, combine the oils, then gradually add the oil to the vinegar mixture, whisking all the while.

To make the salad, in a large bowl, combine all of the vegetables except the lettuce cups.

Pour the dressing over the vegetables, and mix well. Cover, chill, and refrigerate for at least 1 hour.

Divide the salad among the lettuce cups, if desired, and serve.

YIELD: 6 servings   SERVING SIZE: ½ cup

Calories	Protein	Carbohydrates	Fat	Sodium
39	1 g	3 g	3 g	11 mg

Exchange: 1 vegetable; ½ fat

Spinach, Tomato, and Red Onion Salad

This is a delicious salad, with a very strong, almost hot, flavor from the horseradish. If you are in the least sensitive about the "heat" in foods, cut down on the horseradish.

4 cups packed, washed, stemmed, and drained fresh spinach leaves, coarsely chopped

2 ripe medium tomatoes, cut into ¼-inch slices

2 small red onions, halved lengthwise and thinly sliced

½ teaspoon salt, optional

1 tablespoon extra-virgin olive oil

1½ tablespoons balsamic or aged red wine vinegar

2 tablespoons water

½ teaspoon ground white pepper

1½ teaspoons prepared horseradish

1 tablespoon chopped fresh parsley for garnish

Arrange the spinach on a platter or in a large shallow bowl. Place the tomatoes over the spinach and then arrange the onions over the tomatoes. If desired, sprinkle the salt over all of the vegetables.

In a small bowl, whisk together the oil, vinegar, water, white pepper, and horseradish until thoroughly blended. Pour the dressing over the vegetables, garnish with the parsley, and serve.

YIELD: 4 servings   SERVING SIZE: ⅔ cup

Calories	Protein	Carbohydrates	Fat	Sodium
64	3 g	7 g	4 g	49 mg

Exchange: 1 vegetable; 1 fat

Dilled Cucumber Salad

This simple cucumber salad is quick to make and delicious with Poached Salmon (page 282) and other fish dishes or on its own. It requires about 1 hour in the refrigerator before serving.

2 large cucumbers, peeled, seeded, and finely chopped
1 tablespoon white wine vinegar
½ teaspoon salt
½ teaspoon coarsely ground black pepper

½ cup plain nonfat yogurt
1 tablespoon fresh dill, or 1 teaspoon dried, crumbled
1 teaspoon fresh lime or lemon juice
1 teaspoon granulated garlic or garlic powder

In a large bowl, combine the cucumbers, vinegar, salt, and pepper and set aside. In another large bowl, mix the yogurt with the dill, lime juice, and granulated garlic. Fold the cucumber mixture into the yogurt and refrigerate at least 1 hour before serving.

YIELD: 4 servings   SERVING SIZE: ½ to ⅔ cup

Calories	Protein	Carbohydrates	Fat	Sodium
17	0.5 g	2.85 g	0 g	39.25 mg

Exchange: 1 vegetable

Persian Cucumber Salad

This salad should be made with fresh mint leaves only and needs to be refrigerated for about 45 minutes before serving.

*3 large cucumbers, peeled, seeded,
and cut into ¼-by-3½-inch sticks*

*10 to 12 fresh mint leaves, rubbed
with your fingers and then finely
chopped*

Scant ¼ cup minced garlic

*1 medium red bell pepper, stemmed,
seeded, and julienned*

*1 small yellow or white onion,
halved lengthwise and thinly sliced*

*6 large ripe black olives, pitted and
slivered, optional*

¼ cup plain nonfat yogurt

*2 teaspoons fresh lime or lemon
juice*

*Coarsely ground black pepper to
taste*

¼ teaspoon salt, optional

*4 romaine lettuce leaves, cut into
1-inch strips*

In a large bowl, combine the cucumbers, mint, garlic, bell pepper, onion, olives, if desired, yogurt, lime juice, pepper, and salt, if desired. Do this gently to avoid bruising the cucumbers. Refrigerate for about 45 minutes. Divide the lettuce among 6 plates and spoon the cucumber salad over the lettuce.

YIELD: 6 servings   SERVING SIZE: ½ to ⅔ cup

Calories	Protein	Carbohydrates	Fat	Sodium
35	1 g	5 g	1 g	47 mg

Exchange: 1 vegetable

Barley, Cucumber, and Tomato Salad with Yogurt Dressing

This recipe takes about 30 minutes for the barley to cook and about 3 hours in the refrigerator to chill. It can be made in the morning and served that night.

¾ cup pearl barley, thoroughly rinsed

1½ teaspoons mustard seeds

⅓ cup plain nonfat yogurt

2 tablespoons low-fat sour cream or sour cream substitute

1 tablespoon extra-virgin olive oil

3 tablespoons minced fresh dill, or 2 teaspoons dried, crumbled

2 teaspoons granulated garlic or garlic powder

3 large ripe plum tomatoes, cut into medium dice

1 large cucumber, peeled, halved lengthwise, seeded, and thinly sliced

2 green onions, thinly sliced

¼ cup finely chopped red onion

10 ripe black olives, pitted and slivered, optional

Coarsely ground black pepper to taste, optional

Pour the barley into 4 cups of boiling water. Return to a boil and simmer until the barley is tender. This should take about 30 minutes. Drain the barley well and let cool in a large glass bowl.

Meanwhile, toast the mustard seeds by heating them in a medium-hot, dry skillet and shaking the pan until the seeds pop. In a small bowl, mix the yogurt, sour cream, oil, dill, granulated garlic, and toasted mustard seeds. Set aside.

Add the tomatoes, cucumber, green and red onions, and olives, if desired, to the barley. Toss, add the yogurt mixture, and toss again. Add the pepper, if desired. Cover and chill for at least 3 hours.

YIELD: 8 servings   SERVING SIZE: ½ cup

Calories	Protein	Carbohydrates	Fat	Sodium
111	3 g	18 g	3 g	41 mg

Exchange: 1 starch; ½ fat

Mediterranean Salad

This dish requires the oranges and the onion to marinate in the vinaigrette for at least 3 hours or longer. Serve in lettuce cups.

2 teaspoons extra-virgin olive oil

1 teaspoon canola oil

Grated zest and juice of 1 lime

3 tablespoons balsamic or aged red wine vinegar

Coarsely ground black pepper to taste

5 medium garlic cloves, minced

½ teaspoon Dijon-style mustard (substitute a pinch of dry mustard if you prefer)

1 tablespoon sugar substitute

2 large navel or Valencia oranges or tangelos, or 3 tangerines

1 small red onion, halved lengthwise and thinly sliced

16 Bibb or green-leaf lettuce leaves, washed and crisped

In a small bowl, whisk together all of the ingredients except the oranges, onion, and lettuce.

Peel the oranges, section them, and slice the sections into ¼-inch wedges. In a separate bowl, gently toss the onion and oranges, cover them with the vinaigrette, and toss again. Cover and refrigerate for at least 3 hours and up to 24.

Just before serving, form 4 of the lettuce leaves into lettuce cups (see headnote, page 190, for technique). Repeat this procedure with the remaining leaves to form a total of 4 lettuce cups. Divide the marinated orange mixture equally among the lettuce cups.

YIELD: 4 servings   SERVING SIZE: ½ cup

Calories	Protein	Carbohydrates	Fat	Sodium
73	1 g	10 g	3.5 g	16 mg

Exchange: ½ fruit; ½ vegetable; ½ fat

Greek Salad

1 large garlic clove, peeled

1 small head of Bibb or Boston
    lettuce, washed, drained, and
    leaves torn

2 ounces low-fat feta cheese,
    crumbled

2 teaspoons extra-virgin olive oil

3 large ripe plum tomatoes, quartered

1 large cucumber, peeled, seeded, and
    diced

10 small ripe black olives, pitted and
    finely diced

2 tablespoons red wine vinegar

Coarsely ground black pepper to
    taste

Rub the salad bowl with the garlic. Line the bowl with the lettuce. Combine the feta cheese and oil in another bowl. Very gently toss the tomatoes, cucumber, and olives with the feta cheese. Add the vinegar and pepper and turn into the salad bowl. Toss and serve.

YIELD: 4 servings

SERVING SIZE: ½ cup

Calories	Protein	Carbohydrates	Fat	Sodium
102	3 g	5 g	6 g	180 mg

Exchange: 1 vegetable; 1 fat

Vegetable Salad with Feta Cheese

Salad

1 large head of Boston lettuce, or 2
    small heads of Bibb, washed,
    drained, and shredded
2 large carrots, peeled and julienned
    into 2-inch sticks
1 medium green bell pepper,
    stemmed, seeded, and julienned
    into 2-inch sticks
1 (14½-ounce) can sliced beets,
    julienned, or 3 beets, boiled,
    peeled, and julienned
1 large cucumber, peeled, seeded, and
    coarsely chopped
2 large ripe tomatoes, cut into ½-
    inch chunks

1 (14½-ounce) can wax beans
4 large radishes, thinly sliced
1 medium head of radicchio,
    shredded
1 medium head of curly endive,
    thinly sliced
1½ cups fresh or frozen green
    peas
1 small chunk (about 3 inches
    square) jicama, peeled and
    julienned into 2-inch sticks
2 ounces low-fat feta cheese,
    crumbled

Dressing

3 tablespoons balsamic vinegar
1 tablespoon Dijon-style mustard
2 teaspoons extra-virgin olive oil
2 teaspoons canola oil
2½ tablespoons water

Coarsely ground black pepper to
    taste
1 teaspoon minced garlic
Sliced fresh basil leaves for
    garnish

To make the salad, place the lettuce on a serving platter. Arrange all of the vegetables and the feta cheese in separate rows on top of the lettuce.

To make the dressing, whisk together all of the ingredients except the basil in a medium bowl. Sprinkle the dressing over the salad, garnish with the basil, and serve.

YIELD: 6 servings   SERVING SIZE: ½ cup

Calories	Protein	Carbohydrates	Fat	Sodium
164	7 g	21 g	5 g	297 mg

Exchange: 1 starch; 1 vegetable; 1 fat

Lentil Salad

I always use arugula for this salad when it is available; if I cannot get it, I use curly endive or any other strong-tasting green.

1 cup dried lentils (blond, red, or brown)
1 tablespoon canola oil
1 tablespoon balsamic or aged red wine vinegar
2 tablespoons water
¼ teaspoon dry mustard
Coarsely ground black pepper to taste
1 tablespoon finely sliced fresh basil, or 1 teaspoon dried

1 small red onion, finely diced
1 small red bell pepper, stemmed, seeded, and diced
¼ cup coarsely chopped fresh parsley
1 small bunch of arugula, curly endive, or other strong-tasting green (about 1½ cups), cut or torn into bite-size pieces
½ teaspoon salt, optional
2 large limes

Combine the lentils and 3 cups of water and bring to a boil. Cook, uncovered, until tender, 30 minutes. Red lentils will cook in about 25 minutes. Drain thoroughly.

In a small bowl, whisk together the oil, vinegar, water, mustard, and black pepper. In a large bowl, toss the drained lentils with the dressing. Cover and refrigerate for about an hour.

Meanwhile, in a separate bowl, combine the basil, onion, bell pepper, parsley, and arugula. Set aside.

When the lentils are cold, toss them with the salt, if desired, and the juice of 1 lime. When that mixture is thoroughly incorporated, add the mixed vegetables, toss again, and serve garnished with the remaining lime, cut into wedges.

YIELD: 6 servings   SERVING SIZE: ½ cup

Calories	Protein	Carbohydrates	Fat	Sodium
149	10 g	21 g	2 g	8 mg

Exchange: 1 starch; 1 vegetable; 1 lean meat

Bulgur Wheat Salad (Tabbouleh)

This recipe calls for fresh mint leaves. Dried mint simply does not work. When fresh mint is not available, I substitute the same amount of fresh cilantro leaves. It gives the salad a different taste, but the taste is delicious.

Bulgur needs to be soaked in cold water for about 1 hour, then thoroughly drained before it can be used. Once tossed with the dressing, it should be chilled for about 30 minutes before you finish the salad and serve. It can be chilled all day or overnight.

½ cup bulgur

2 teaspoons extra-virgin olive or
canola oil

1 tablespoon water

½ cup fresh lime or lemon juice

1 teaspoon salt

Coarsely ground black pepper to
taste

¾ cup finely minced fresh parsley

5 tablespoons finely chopped fresh
mint or cilantro leaves

¾ cup finely chopped red onion,
green onions, or scallions

¾ cup diced ripe tomatoes

2 cups thinly sliced romaine lettuce

Lime or lemon wedges for garnish

Soak the bulgur in cold water to cover for about 1 hour. Drain well and press out the excess water. In a large bowl, combine the bulgur with the oil, water, lime juice, salt, pepper, parsley, mint, and onion. Toss, cover, and chill for about 30 minutes.

When you are ready to serve, toss the tomatoes with the bulgur mixture. Divide the lettuce equally among 6 plates and top with the bulgur. Serve garnished with the lime wedges.

YIELD: 6 servings   SERVING SIZE: ½ cup

Calories	Protein	Carbohydrates	Fat	Sodium
85	3 g	16 g	2 g	128 mg

Exchange: 1 starch

Tomatoes Stuffed with Vegetable Pasta Salad

These stuffed tomatoes are delicious but do require a bit of advance work, all of which can be done the night or the morning before. Everything can be held in the refrigerator for 24 hours.

¼ cup orzo or other small pasta

1 very large ear yellow or white
   corn, kernels cut from the cob
   (see instructions, page 218), or
   ½ cup frozen corn kernels,
   thawed

1 large zucchini, sliced

¼ pound fresh green beans, ends
   trimmed

6 large firm, ripe tomatoes

1 recipe Tarragon Dressing (recipe
   follows)

½ cup thinly sliced green onions or
   scallions

Coarsely ground black pepper to
   taste

2 tablespoons finely minced fresh
   parsley

In a medium saucepan with a cover, bring about 3 cups of water to a boil. Add the pasta and cook until just tender to the bite (about 6 or 7 minutes). Drain the pasta, rinse under cold running water, and chill in the refrigerator.

In the same pot, quickly bring a small amount of water to a boil and using a steamer insert, steam the fresh corn, if using, zucchini, and green beans for about 5 minutes. Immediately plunge the vegetables into an ice water bath and when cold, drain. If using thawed frozen corn, add it to the steamed vegetables now. Chill the mixture in the refrigerator.

Cut the tops from the tomatoes about ½ inch down and set aside.

With a spoon, scoop out the insides and either freeze for future use or discard. Drain the tomato cups and chill in the refrigerator.

Chop the tomato tops, cut the zucchini into small dice, and thinly slice the green beans on the diagonal. Mix all of these ingredients in a large bowl with the chilled pasta. All of this can be done up to 24 hours in advance.

When you are ready to serve, combine the pasta mixture with the dressing, green onions, pepper, and parsley. Toss the pasta salad and then fill the tomato cups with it.

Tarragon Dressing

2 teaspoons extra-virgin olive oil
1 teaspoon canola oil
1 tablespoon balsamic vinegar
1 tablespoon cold water

1 teaspoon dried tarragon, or 1½ tablespoons fresh tarragon
1¼ teaspoons Dijon-style mustard
1 large garlic clove, finely minced

In a small bowl, whisk all of the ingredients together and chill. The dressing may be made in advance.

YIELD: 6 servings   SERVING SIZE: 1 stuffed tomato

Calories	Protein	Carbohydrates	Fat	Sodium
107	4 g	16 g	3 g	38 mg

Exchange: 1 starch; ½ fat

Thai Tofu Salad

This salad, which is served hot, also works well as an entrée; chicken can be substituted for the tofu.

Roasted rice powder, used here as a thickening agent, is really easy to make, and you will find yourself using it in other recipes. Thai tofu also uses Sambal Oeleck, a very spicy Thai chili sauce that is available in many supermarkets and all Asian markets.

5 tablespoons fresh lime juice

3 teaspoons fish sauce or reduced- or low-sodium soy sauce

1½ cups Chicken Broth (page 133), Garlic Broth (page 132), Vegetable Broth (page 128), or low-fat, low-sodium canned broth

3 tablespoons minced garlic

3 teaspoons minced fresh ginger

1 teaspoon Sambal Oeleck, or ¼ teaspoon hot chili oil

1 heaping teaspoon granulated sugar substitute

1 tablespoon Roasted Rice Powder (recipe follows)

3 medium serrano chilies, seeded and thinly sliced

1 pound extra-firm tofu, thinly sliced

1 small red onion, halved and French cut across the wedge into thin, uniform slices

½ cup green onions or scallions, cut into 2-inch strips

2 tablespoons chopped fresh mint leaves

¼ cup chopped fresh cilantro leaves

1 large cucumber, peeled, seeded, and cut into ½-inch chunks

2 large ripe tomatoes, cut into eighths

2 cups shredded Napa cabbage, bok choy, or other Chinese cabbage (use regular green cabbage if the others are not available)

2 cups shredded romaine lettuce

2 cups cooked rice for serving

In a large skillet or a wok over medium heat, simmer the lime juice, fish sauce, and broth. Reduce the liquid a bit and add the garlic, ginger, Sambal Oeleck, sugar substitute, rice powder, and chilies. Bring to a boil and add the tofu.

Stir and add the red and green onions and again bring to a boil. Add the mint, cilantro, cucumber, and tomatoes. Stir and add the cabbage and lettuce. Cook 1 minute, toss, and serve over the rice.

YIELD: 4 servings   SERVING SIZE: ¾ cup salad plus ½ cup rice

Roasted Rice Powder

2 tablespoons short- or long-grain white rice

Roast the rice in a toaster oven or in a 450°F oven until it turns golden brown. This will take about 2 minutes in a toaster oven and about 5 minutes in a conventional oven.

Grind the rice in a food mill or food processor. It will keep in an airtight container on the shelf for several months.

YIELD: 2 tablespoons

Calories	Protein	Carbohydrates	Fat	Sodium
227	14 g	34 g	5 g	188 mg

Exchange: 1½ starches; 2 vegetables; 1½ medium-fat meats

Southwestern Chicken Salad

This salad also can be used as an entrée with appropriate side dishes. It can be prepared several hours in advance. If you wish to be able to serve the dish quickly, you need to have cooked, skinless chicken on hand.

1 cup skinless diced cooked chicken

2 large ripe plum tomatoes, diced

1 cucumber, peeled, seeded, and diced

1/4 cup peeled and julienned jicama

1/4 cup peeled and julienned carrot

1/4 cup finely chopped fresh or drained low-sodium canned water chestnuts

1/4 cup finely chopped fresh Anaheim or frozen green chilies

4 green onions, thinly sliced

3 tablespoons fresh lime or lemon juice

1 tablespoon extra-virgin olive oil

1/4 cup minced fresh cilantro leaves

Pinch of salt

Coarsely ground black pepper to taste

1/4 teaspoon dried oregano, crumbled

1 small avocado, peeled and diced, optional

2 cups shredded romaine or green-leaf lettuce

Lime wedges for garnish

In a large bowl, combine the chicken, tomatoes, cucumber, jicama, carrot, water chestnuts, chilies, green onions, lime juice, oil, and cilantro. Season with the salt, pepper, and oregano and mix thoroughly.

Gently fold the avocado, if desired, into the salad and serve on beds of lettuce. Garnish with the lime wedges and serve.

YIELD: 6 servings   SERVING SIZE: ⅔ cup

Calories	Protein	Carbohydrates	Fat	Sodium
113	8 g	6 g	6 g	26 mg

Exchange: 1 vegetable; 1 lean meat; 1 fat

Crunchy Chicken Salad

This recipe tastes best if the chicken has been precooked and chilled. The chicken salad can then be put together quickly and will stay very crunchy.

1½ to 2 cups skinless chopped cooked chicken

1 small red bell pepper, stemmed, seeded, and diced

½ cup sliced fresh or drained low-sodium canned water chestnuts, chilled

¼ cup toasted sliced almonds

1 cup diced celery

2 tablespoons fresh lime or lemon juice

¼ cup low-fat, no-cholesterol mayonnaise (eggless mayonnaise is available at most markets)

2 tablespoons plain nonfat yogurt

2 tablespoons minced fresh parsley

Coarsely ground black pepper to taste

¼ teaspoon salt substitute, optional

In a large bowl, mix the chicken, bell pepper, water chestnuts, almonds, celery, lime juice, mayonnaise, yogurt, and parsley. Season with the pepper and salt substitute, if desired. Toss to combine thoroughly. Serve.

YIELD: 6 servings   SERVING SIZE: ½ cup

Calories	Protein	Carbohydrates	Fat	Sodium
133	14 g	6 g	6 g	182 mg

Exchange: 2 lean meats; ½ starch

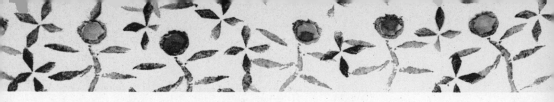

Vegetables and Side Dishes

Lemon Broccoli

Brussels Sprout Sauté with Apples
and Onions

"Creamed" Corn

Baked Corn

Herbed Soybean Casserole

Green Beans with Mustard and Ginger

Spinach Sauté

Eggplant Parmesan

Sautéed Asian Eggplant with Snow Peas

Stuffed Acorn Squash

Barley-Mushroom Pilaf

Roasted Sliced Potatoes

New Potatoes with Turmeric and Cumin

Sweet Potato and Apple Scallop

Skillet Creamed Potatoes

Curried Potatoes

Lyonnaise Potatoes

Spicy Sweet Potato Fritters

Lemon Broccoli

Simple and delicious.

1 large bunch of broccoli
Juice of 1 large lemon or lime

Rinse the broccoli thoroughly, separate the florets from the stems, and chop the stems.

Pour ½ cup of water into a medium saucepan and insert a steamer. Cover and bring the water to a boil. Add the stems, cover, and steam for about 3 minutes. Uncover and stir the stems. Place the florets on top, cover, and steam for another 3 minutes. Serve with the lemon juice.

To cook in the microwave, place the broccoli stems in a glass bowl with about 2 tablespoons of water and cover loosely with plastic wrap. Poke several holes in the wrap and microwave the stems on high for about 2 minutes. Add the florets, put in another tablespoon of water, re-cover, and cook for another 2 minutes. Serve with the lemon juice.

YIELD: 6 servings   SERVING SIZE: ½ cup

Calories	Protein	Carbohydrates	Fat	Sodium
26	2.4 g	5.2 g	0.2 g	20 mg

Exchange: 1 vegetable

VARIATIONS

Lemon Cauliflower: Separate 1 head of cauliflower into florets. Using the same amount of water, steam in the same manner for 3 or 4 minutes. To microwave, use 1 tablespoon of water and cook on high for 3 minutes 15 seconds. Serve with the lemon juice.

Lemon Carrots: Peel and slice 3 large carrots into ⅛- to ¼-inch pieces. Using the same amount of water, steam in the same manner for about 3 minutes. To microwave, use 1 tablespoon of water and cook on high for 3 to 3½ minutes. Serve with the lemon juice.

Lemon Zucchini or Yellow Crookneck Squash: Pare the tips of 3 medium squash and slice into ¼-inch pieces. Using the same amount of water, steam in the same manner for about 3 minutes. To microwave, use 1 tablespoon of water and cook on high for about 1½ minutes. Serve with the lemon juice.

Brussels Sprout Sauté with Apples and Onions

A great winter vegetable idea. The dish is simple to make, very flavorful, and a wonderful accompaniment to chicken.

¾ pound brussels sprouts, trimmed and halved

2 teaspoons canola oil

1 small yellow onion, cut into medium dice

1½ cups cored and thinly sliced red apples (Gala or Red Delicious)

1 teaspoon dried marjoram, crumbled

½ teaspoon dried thyme, crumbled

½ teaspoon salt substitute

Scant teaspoon ground white pepper

Bring 4 cups of water to a boil in a heavy 2-quart saucepan. Add the brussels sprouts, cover, and cook for 4 to 6 minutes. At this point they should be tender. Drain and set aside.

In a large (10- or 12-inch) skillet over medium heat, heat the oil. Add the onion and cook for 4 to 5 minutes, stirring frequently, until the onion is softened. Add the apples and stir. Cook until the apples are lightly browned and just barely tender (about 5 minutes).

Add the brussels sprouts along with the herbs, salt substitute, and white pepper. Continue cooking for about 4 minutes more, until everything is thoroughly heated. As you cook, toss the mixture to make sure that it is combined. Serve.

YIELD: **4 servings**   SERVING SIZE: ¾ cup

Calories	Protein	Carbohydrates	Fat	Sodium
88	2.5 g	15.5 g	2.81 g	17.25 mg

Exchange: 1 vegetable; ½ fruit; ½ fat

"Creamed" Corn

For this dish, fresh corn must be used, as the "cream" in the creamed corn comes from the cob itself. This is a very simple dish to prepare, and when corn is in season, it is also inexpensive. It is one you will love to have again and again.

4 large ears fresh corn
Nonstick cooking spray for sautéing
1 small yellow or white onion, cut into small dice
½ cup finely diced red bell pepper
½ cup Chicken Broth (page 133), Vegetable Broth (page 128), or low-fat, low-sodium canned broth

Salt substitute to taste
Coarsely ground black pepper to taste
¼ teaspoon ground nutmeg
1 tablespoon minced fresh parsley or chives for garnish

Remove the husks and the silk from the corn. Place the base of the corn in a deep bowl or pot and with a sharp knife, cut the kernels from the tip of the cob to the base. Be sure not to cut down too deeply into the cob, as you will need the pulp later and don't want any of the tough fibers mixed in.

Heat a medium skillet over medium heat, lightly coat it with the nonstick cooking spray, and add the, corn, onion, and bell pepper. Sauté until the onion is softened and then pour in the broth. Add the salt substitute, black pepper, and nutmeg. Cover and simmer for 5 to 6 minutes.

Into the same bowl you used to remove the kernels, scrape the pulp from each cob by running a sharp knife tip lengthwise down the center of each row of corn (the imprint of each row will still be visible on the cob) and then turning the blade over to the blunt side and firmly running it down the cob to release the milky juices and the pulp. Put all of the pulp in the skillet with the vegetable sauté.

Mix well and continue to cook until the corn is tender. Garnish with the parsley and serve.

YIELD: 4 servings   SERVING SIZE: ½ cup

Calories	Protein	Carbohydrates	Fat	Sodium
101	3.5 g	22.38 g	1 g	14.38 mg

Exchange: 1½ starches

Baked Corn

Nonstick cooking spray for the pie
  tin and sautéing

6 medium ears fresh corn, or 3 cups
  frozen corn, thawed

3 shallots, finely minced, or 5
  tablespoons finely minced white
  onion

1 small red bell pepper, stemmed,
  seeded, and finely diced

The equivalent of 3 eggs in egg
  substitute, or 3 eggs

½ teaspoon salt substitute

Coarsely ground black pepper to
  taste

1½ teaspoons granulated garlic or
  garlic powder

3 tablespoons minced fresh parsley

Preheat the oven to 350°F. Lightly coat 1 (9-inch) pie tin or 4 (3-inch) tart rings with the nonstick cooking spray.

Cut the corn kernels from the cobs (see instructions, page 218) or drain the thawed frozen corn. Heat a large skillet over medium heat and lightly coat it with the cooking spray. Toss in the shallots and sauté until soft. Add the bell pepper and corn. Cook the mixture until the bell pepper is somewhat softened.

Meanwhile, in a large bowl, beat the eggs thoroughly with the salt substitute, black pepper, and granulated garlic. Add the vegetable sauté, combine, and turn the whole mixture into the pie tin(s) and bake until just set in the center, 30 to 40 minutes.

Serve hot or at room temperature and garnish with the parsley.

YIELD: 6 servings   SERVING SIZE: ½ cup

Calories	*Protein*	*Carbohydrates*	*Fat*	*Sodium*
104.83	5.32 g	22.23 g	1.05 g	48 mg

Exchange: 1½ starches

Herbed Soybean Casserole

Unlike the rest of the pea family, the soybean (or soya bean, as it is also known) is high in protein and low in carbohydrates. It is nutritious, has a bland taste, and readily absorbs the flavors of stronger-tasting foods. In many cultures it is used as a substitute for meat. Tofu (a Japanese term for a Chinese discovery) is made from the soybean and has become a very popular source of protein in the United States. When served with a salad or a vegetable, this dish can easily be used as an entrée.

I use dried soybeans to make this casserole. There are two easy methods of preparing the beans so that they will be tender enough to cook: (1) You can put the dried beans in a large pot or bowl, cover them with cool water, and let them soak overnight, or (2) you can put the dried beans in a large pot, cover them with cool water, bring them to a boil, and boil them for 5 minutes. Then put a lid on the pot, remove the pot from the stove, and let the beans rest for 1 hour.

Either method works, but the soaking overnight is simpler if you have the time. Whichever method you use, you must then cook the beans for about 2 hours before they are ready to use.

All of this can be done in advance, and you can refrigerate the soybeans for several days or freeze them for future use. You may use canned beans if you wish. However you store them, be sure to save the liquid in which they cook.

³/₄ cup dried soybeans (2 cups cooked)

2 small bay leaves

Nonstick cooking spray for sautéing

1 small yellow onion, finely minced

1 tablespoon finely minced garlic

1 teaspoon dried dill, crumbled

2 tablespoons minced fresh parsley, or 1 teaspoon dried, crumbled

Coarsely ground black pepper to taste

2 tablespoons grated low-fat Parmesan cheese

3 ripe medium tomatoes, cut into ¼-inch slices

3 medium yellow crookneck squash, thinly sliced

½ teaspoon paprika, optional

Soak the beans according to method 1 or 2 (see headnote), then drain them. Place the beans, bay leaves, and 3 to 4 cups of water in a large pot over high heat. Bring to a boil, reduce the heat, and cook for 2 hours, until the beans are tender. Drain the beans, reserving about ¾ cup of the cooking liquid. Discard the bay leaves.

Heat a large skillet over medium heat, lightly coat with the nonstick cooking spray, and sauté the onion for several minutes. Add the garlic, dill, parsley, and pepper and sauté for several minutes more.

Add the beans and their cooking liquid and simmer, uncovered, in the skillet for about 15 minutes.

Preheat the oven to 350°F and lightly coat a 3-quart ovenproof casserole dish with the cooking spray.

Add the Parmesan cheese to the beans and thoroughly stir. Pour half of the bean mixture into the prepared casserole. Cover the beans with a layer of tomatoes, and then cover the tomatoes with a layer of squash. Repeat the layers: beans, tomatoes, squash.

Sprinkle with the paprika, if desired, cover, and bake for 1 to 1¼ hours. Serve hot.

YIELD: 4 servings   SERVING SIZE: ⅔ cup

Calories	Protein	Carbohydrates	Fat	Sodium
195	13.73 g	17.75 g	7.5 g	40.5 mg

Exchange: 1 lean meat; 1 starch; 1½ fats

Green Beans with Mustard and Ginger

This dish is as good served cold or at room temperature as it is served hot. I prefer harvester beans — the round ones — as their taste is more delicate, they are not tough, and they are easy to obtain all year.

3 teaspoons Dijon-style mustard
3 teaspoons balsamic or aged red
    wine vinegar
2 heaping teaspoons minced fresh
    ginger
¼ teaspoon salt substitute
Coarsely ground black pepper to
    taste

¼ teaspoon cayenne pepper
½ teaspoon granulated garlic or
    garlic powder
2 teaspoons canola oil
1 teaspoon extra-virgin olive oil
1 pound fresh green beans, stem
    ends trimmed

In a 3-quart pot, bring ½ gallon of water to a boil over high heat.

Meanwhile, put the mustard in a small bowl and then whisk in the vinegar, ginger, salt substitute, black pepper, cayenne pepper, and the granulated garlic. Combine the oils and add them to the mustard mixture as you continue to whisk it rapidly.

Drop the beans into the boiling water and boil rapidly for 4 to 5 minutes, until the beans are tender-crisp.

Pull the beans immediately from the water and thoroughly drain. Put the beans into a serving dish and toss with the dressing. Serve.

YIELD: 4 servings   SERVING SIZE: ½ cup

Calories	Protein	Carbohydrates	Fat	Sodium
70	2 g	8 g	4 g	93 mg

Exchange: 1 vegetable; 1 fat

Spinach Sauté

When fresh spinach is used, it is very important to make sure that the spinach is thoroughly washed and dried. I find that the easiest way to dry spinach is with paper towels or with a salad spinner.

2 teaspoons extra-virgin olive oil

¼ cup diced yellow onion

3 medium garlic cloves, minced

Coarsely ground black pepper to taste

2 teaspoons dried dill, crumbled

2 bunches of spinach (about 2 pounds) thoroughly washed, stemmed, and drained

½ cup plain nonfat yogurt

1 teaspoon sesame seeds, optional

3 tablespoons freshly grated Parmesan cheese

1 tablespoon minced fresh parsley

Heat a large skillet over medium heat, add the oil, and sauté the onion, garlic, pepper, and dill for several minutes. Add the spinach and sauté lightly until wilted (about 5 minutes).

Add the yogurt and heat until the mixture is thoroughly warmed. Sprinkle with the sesame seeds, if desired, Parmesan cheese, and parsley. Serve.

YIELD: 6 servings   SERVING SIZE: ½ cup

Calories	Protein	Carbohydrates	Fat	Sodium
46.5	3.38 g	3.42 g	3.61 g	134.6 mg

Exchange: ¼ milk; 1 vegetable; ½ fat

Eggplant Parmesan

This is another side dish that also works well as an entrée.

1 large or 2 small firm and
  unblemished eggplants, unpeeled
2 teaspoons extra-virgin olive oil
2 teaspoons coarsely ground black
  pepper
2 teaspoons granulated garlic or
  garlic powder

2 cups Marinara Sauce (page 171)
  or Jiffy Marinara Sauce (page
  173)
¼ cup low-fat Parmesan cheese
2 tablespoons finely minced fresh
  parsley for garnish

Preheat the oven to 400°F.

Cut the large eggplant into 12 slices or the small ones into 6 slices each. Oil a cookie sheet with 1 teaspoon of the oil and place the eggplant slices in a single layer on the sheet. Sprinkle them with half of the pepper and granulated garlic.

Bake until the eggplant slices are lightly browned (about 8 minutes) and turn them over. Sprinkle with the remaining pepper and granulated garlic and cook about 7 minutes more.

Meanwhile, heat the marinara sauce and lower the oven to 300°F.

Oil the bottoms of 4 individual casserole dishes or that of 1 large casserole dish with the remaining oil. Place the eggplant in the oiled dishes in a single layer.

Ladle ½ cup of the warmed sauce over the eggplant in each individual dish or pour the whole 2 cups of the sauce on top of the eggplant in the large baking dish. Sprinkle 1 tablespoon of the cheese on top of the sauce-covered eggplant in each individual dish, or sprinkle the entire amount on top of the sauce-covered eggplant in the large dish.

Put the dishes in the oven and heat until the cheese melts. Top with the parsley and serve.

YIELD: 4 servings   SERVING SIZE: 3 slices of eggplant

Calories	Protein	Carbohydrates	Fat	Sodium
95.38	3.13 g	10.29 g	4.05 g	134.25 mg

Exchange: ½ medium-fat meat; 2 vegetables; 1 fat

Sautéed Asian Eggplant with Snow Peas

This is one of those dishes you will want to cook over and over again. It is simple to make, delicious, and visually appealing. This can easily be cooked in a skillet, but a wok or stir-fry pan works best.

If you want to use the eggplant as an entrée, serve over rice or Chinese noodles and add a dish that is complementary protein-wise, such as tofu or soybeans.

2 purple Asian eggplants, or 1 medium eggplant, unpeeled and cut into 1-inch cubes

¼ cup minced garlic

1 large yellow or white onion, cut into medium dice

2 tablespoons reduced- or low-sodium soy sauce

2 tablespoons brown sugar substitute

1 teaspoon hot chili oil (available at Asian and many local markets)

2 teaspoons cornstarch dissolved in ⅓ cup cold water

½ cup finely chopped red bell pepper

1 cup fresh snow peas, trimmed

½ cup drained sliced low-sodium canned water chestnuts

½ cup sliced green onions or scallions

In a large skillet or wok over medium-high heat, bring 1 cup of water to a boil. Put in the eggplant. Add the garlic, yellow onion, soy sauce, brown sugar substitute, and chili oil to the eggplant and cook, partially covered, until the eggplant is tender.

If you are using a skillet rather than a wok, push the vegetables to one side so that the liquid in the pan is easily visible. If you are using a wok, push the vegetables up the side of the pan so that you can easily get to the liquid. Stir in the dissolved cornstarch.

Cook the liquid so it thickens at the same time you add the bell pepper, snow peas, water chestnuts, and green onions. Stir quickly into the vegetable mixture. Thoroughly combine and serve.

YIELD: 4 to 6 servings   SERVING SIZE: ½ to ⅔ cup

Calories	Protein	Carbohydrates	Fat	Sodium
45	1.7 g	8 g	0.8 g	223.9 mg

Exchange: 1½ vegetables

Stuffed Acorn Squash

This side dish can also be served as an entrée, with an appropriate side dish such as tofu or a hearty soup to form a complete protein. You need to cook the rice in advance for this dish. I like to mound any extra rice stuffing in the center of the serving platter with the squash arranged around it. You may also freeze any remaining stuffing for future use.

2 small to medium acorn squash

Nonstick cooking spray for sautéing

⅓ cup diced yellow onion

6 large mushrooms, thinly sliced

1½ tablespoons minced garlic

⅓ cup finely sliced red bell pepper

¾ cup cooked basmati or short- or long-grain brown rice

½ teaspoon dried thyme, crumbled

1 teaspoon dried basil, crumbled

2 teaspoons coarsely ground black pepper

1 teaspoon grated lemon or lime zest

Preheat the oven to 350°F.

Split the squash lengthwise in half, scoop out the seeds and the strings, place the squash halves cut-side down on a baking sheet, and pierce the shells in 3 or 4 places. Bake until the squash is tender, for 25 to 30 minutes.

Meanwhile, heat a medium (8- or 10-inch) skillet over medium heat and lightly coat it with the nonstick cooking spray. Add the onion, mushrooms, garlic, and bell pepper and cook about 3 minutes, until the vegetables are barely softened.

Remove from the heat and toss with the rice, herbs, black pepper, and lemon zest. Spoon one-quarter of the rice mixture into each squash cavity.

Arrange the halves on a baking sheet. Cover and bake for about 20 minutes.

Cut each half in half and serve 8 as a side dish or serve each stuffed squash half as an entrée.

YIELD: 8 servings if used as a side dish; 4 servings if used as an entrée

SERVING SIZE: ¼ squash if used as a side dish; ½ squash if used as an entrée

Calories	Protein	Carbohydrates	Fat	Sodium
75	1.63 g	14.47 g	1.75 g	1.33 mg

(Double the amounts of the nutritional analyses if you serve the squash as an entrée.)

Exchange: 1 starch

Barley-Mushroom Pilaf

Soy flakes used in this recipe are soybeans that have been cooked, split, and dehydrated. They are available at health food stores and add a delicious, nutty flavor to food. You may substitute an equal amount of wheat germ or eliminate the ingredient entirely. Any pilaf left over from this dish makes an excellent stuffing for zucchini. It also reheats nicely and can be frozen for future use.

2 teaspoons extra-virgin olive oil

1 large onion, halved lengthwise and thinly sliced

2 large garlic cloves, minced (if using water rather than broth, use 4 garlic cloves)

1 medium red bell pepper, stemmed, seeded, and cut into medium dice

½ pound mushrooms, sliced

2 celery stalks, finely diced

1½ tablespoons dry white wine, optional

2 teaspoons dried basil, crumbled

3 cups Chicken Broth (page 133), Vegetable Broth (page 128), low-fat, low-sodium canned broth, or water

1½ cups barley, rinsed and drained

⅓ cup soy flakes

3 teaspoons coarsely ground black pepper

2 teaspoons dried dill, crumbled

2 tablespoons finely minced fresh parsley for garnish

Preheat the oven to 350°F.

In a large ovenproof casserole or Dutch oven, heat the oil and sauté the onion and half of the garlic until the onion is soft. Add the bell pepper, mushrooms, celery, and remaining garlic. Sauté for about 2 minutes more. Add the wine, if desired, and basil. Sauté for 1 minute more.

Meanwhile, in another pot, bring the broth to a low boil.

Stir the barley and the boiling broth into the vegetable sauté. Add the soy flakes, black pepper, and dill and bring to a boil. Stir, cover, and place the casserole in the oven.

Bake for 30 to 35 minutes, until the barley is tender. Check during the baking to see that the liquid in the pilaf has not evaporated before the barley is tender. If it has, add about ⅓ cup more liquid (water is fine, or more broth if you have it) and continue cooking.

Garnish with the parsley and serve.

YIELD: 4 to 6 servings   SERVING SIZE: ½ cup

Calories	Protein	Carbohydrates	Fat	Sodium
122	6 g	19 g	2 g	16 mg

Exchange: 1 starch; 1 vegetable; ½ fat

Roasted Sliced Potatoes

The potatoes can be sliced ahead of time. Scrub them, cut them into ¼-inch slices, and put them into cold water until you are ready to cook. Then drain and thoroughly blot the slices dry.

1½ tablespoons extra-virgin olive or canola oil

1½ teaspoons granulated garlic or garlic powder

Dash of salt substitute

Ground white pepper to taste

½ to 1 teaspoon dried rosemary, crumbled

2 large baking potatoes, unpeeled, thoroughly scrubbed, and cut into ¼-inch slices

Preheat the oven to 400°F.

In a small bowl, combine the oil, granulated garlic, salt substitute, white pepper, and rosemary. Transfer the oil mixture to one side of a baking sheet. Be sure to scrape all of the mixture out of the bowl, as you will need it.

Rub both sides of each potato slice in the oil mixture and place on the sheet. When you have done this to all of the slices, put the baking sheet on the top shelf of the oven.

Bake for about 15 minutes and then remove the sheet from the oven and turn the slices over. Bake for an additional 10 minutes. The potatoes should be golden brown and tender. Serve.

YIELD: 4 servings

SERVING SIZE: ½ cup; 3 to 4 slices

Calories	Protein	Carbohydrates	Fat	Sodium
135	1.5 g	17 g	5.25 g	4 mg

Exchange: 1 starch; 1 fat

VARIATION

Roasted New Potatoes: Substitute 8 to 12 small new potatoes and use the same amount of oil, granulated garlic, and salt substitute. Omit the ground white pepper and the rosemary. Add ½ teaspoon coarsely ground black pepper, ½ teaspoon paprika, and 1 tablespoon minced fresh parsley. Mix all of the ingredients except for the parsley and the potatoes. Cut the potatoes in half and oil and season the cut sides. Roast in a 400°F oven for 17 to 20 minutes with the cut sides down, turn over, and roast 8 to 10 minutes more. Sprinkle with the parsley and serve.

YIELD: 4 servings   SERVING SIZE: ½ cup; 4 potato halves

Calories	Protein	Carbohydrates	Fat	Sodium
104	1 g	13.5 g	5.25 g	4 mg

Exchange: 1 starch; 1 fat

New Potatoes with Turmeric and Cumin

The potatoes for this dish need to be parboiled before they are sautéed with the spices. If you have the potatoes cooked the night or the morning before, then putting the dish together is quite fast.

16 small (1-inch) new or red
  potatoes
2 teaspoons extra-virgin olive or
  canola oil
1 teaspoon cumin seeds
¼ teaspoon ground turmeric
1 tablespoon low-fat margarine, cut
  into small pieces

1 teaspoon granulated garlic or
  garlic powder
Coarsely ground black pepper to
  taste
Dash of cayenne pepper, optional
½ teaspoon salt substitute
1 tablespoon minced fresh
  parsley

Boil the potatoes in their skins until they are done. Thoroughly drain and cool.

Heat the oil in a large skillet or wok over medium heat until the oil is hot. Add the cumin seeds and then immediately add the turmeric. Lower the heat and stir in the margarine.

Toss in the potatoes, granulated garlic, black pepper, cayenne pepper, if desired, and salt substitute. Stir the potatoes in the skillet for several minutes until hot. Toss in the parsley and serve.

YIELD: 4 servings   SERVING SIZE: 4 potatoes

Calories	Protein	Carbohydrates	Fat	Sodium
92	1 g	15 g	4 g	20 mg

Exchange: 1 starch; ½ fat

Sweet Potato and Apple Scallop

This dish uses baked sweet potatoes. I find it much easier to bake the sweet potatoes in advance and refrigerate them until I'm ready to use them.

Nonstick cooking spray for the
 baking dish
2 medium sweet potatoes, baked,
 peeled, and thinly sliced (about 2
 cups)
1½ cups peeled, cored, and thinly
 sliced tart apples (Granny
 Smith, Gala, or Newton)

⅓ cup brown sugar substitute
2 tablespoons low-fat margarine
Salt substitute to taste

Preheat the oven to 350°F. Lightly coat a 1½-quart baking dish with the nonstick cooking spray.

Layer half of the sweet potatoes in the bottom of the baking dish. Cover the potatoes with half of the apples. Sprinkle with half of the brown sugar substitute and dot with half of the margarine. Sprinkle with the salt substitute. Repeat the layers — potatoes, apples, brown sugar substitute, salt substitute — dotting with the margarine to finish.

Cover and bake for 30 minutes. Uncover and bake for another 20 minutes, or until the apples are soft. Serve hot.

YIELD: 4 servings   SERVING SIZE: ½ cup

Calories	Protein	Carbohydrates	Fat	Sodium
96.46	0.67 g	13.33 g	4.27 g	3.67 mg

Exchange: 1 starch; ½ fat

Skillet Creamed Potatoes

A fast and easy way to have "creamy" potatoes without the fat and without having to bake the potatoes in the oven and heat up the kitchen. I don't usually peel my potatoes, but you may if you wish.

6 (about 1¼ pounds) medium-large
  new potatoes
1 small onion, halved lengthwise
  and thinly sliced
Salt substitute to taste

⅓ cup 1% milk
Coarsely ground black pepper to
  taste
½ teaspoon dried dill, optional
2 tablespoons minced fresh parsley

Thoroughly scrub the potatoes and pat dry with a paper towel. Cut the potatoes into thin slices either by hand or in a food processor.

Meanwhile, heat ½ cup of water to boiling. If any of the water evaporates, add more, as you must have ½ cup of boiling water. (It helps to have a kettle on hand so that you can measure the water after it comes to a boil.)

Heat a large skillet and put in the potatoes and onion. Cover them with the boiling water and a sprinkle of salt substitute. Cover the skillet and braise over medium heat for 6 to 8 minutes. Uncover and cook until the water evaporates. Lower the heat.

Add the milk, pepper, and dill, if desired. Cook, uncovered, over low heat until the potatoes are done and the mixture is slightly thickened. Sprinkle with the parsley and serve.

YIELD: 4 servings   SERVING SIZE: ½ cup

Calories	Protein	Carbohydrates	Fat	Sodium
77	1.9 g	16.49 g	0.41 g	15.50 mg

Exchange: 1 starch

Curried Potatoes

This dish requires cooked, peeled, and diced potatoes. Bake or boil the potatoes in advance, refrigerate them, and peel them when they are cold.

2 teaspoons extra-virgin olive oil

1 small yellow onion, finely diced

3 medium potatoes, cooked, peeled, and cut into medium dice (about 2 cups)

½ cup Chicken Broth (page 133), Garlic Broth (page 132), Vegetable Broth (page 128), or low-fat, low-sodium canned broth

2 teaspoons good-quality curry powder

2 teaspoons fresh lime or lemon juice

Salt substitute to taste

Ground white pepper to taste

In a large skillet over medium heat, heat the oil, toss in the onion, and sauté until the onion is transparent.

Lower the heat, add the potatoes, and sauté, stirring occasionally, until the potatoes absorb all of the oil.

Add the broth, curry powder, and lime juice. Sprinkle with the salt substitute and white pepper. Stir to blend, and braise until all of the broth is absorbed. Serve.

YIELD: 4 servings   SERVING SIZE: ½ cup

Calories	Protein	Carbohydrates	Fat	Sodium
109	1.75 g	19 g	2.34 g	4.50 mg

Exchange: 1 starch; ½ fat

Lyonnaise Potatoes

This is a fairly quick dish and is certainly easy to make. The flavor of the beef stock with the potatoes is delicious and gives you the taste sensation of having potatoes smothered in rich gravy without all of the work, fat, and salt.

The potatoes can be cut up in advance if they are immediately put in cold water. Drain and pat dry before using.

2 teaspoons canola oil
1 small onion, finely chopped
2½ cups peeled and cubed
　potatoes
½ teaspoon coarsely ground black
　pepper

½ teaspoon granulated garlic or
　garlic powder
¼ cup Beef Broth (page 135) or
　low-fat, low-sodium canned broth
1 tablespoon finely minced fresh
　chives or parsley

In a large skillet over medium heat, heat the oil and sauté the onion until it starts to become transparent. Add the potatoes and thoroughly mix them with the onion. Add the pepper and the granulated garlic. Stir in the broth, lower the heat to a simmer, and cover the skillet. Periodically stir the potatoes and continue cooking until the potatoes are tender and browned. Sprinkle the chives over all and serve.

YIELD: 4 servings   SERVING SIZE: ½ cup

Calories	Protein	Carbohydrates	Fat	Sodium
90	2 g	16.5 g	2.34 g	3.75 mg

Exchange: 1 starch; ½ fat

Spicy Sweet Potato Fritters

Unlike most fritters, which are dipped in batter and then deep-fried, these potato "fritters" are lightly coated with a thin batter that forms a crisp shell and then browned with a very small amount of nonstick cooking spray or in a nonstick pan. The sweet potatoes need first to be cooked in the microwave (according to the manufacturer's instructions) or baked in a 450°F oven for about 1 hour, cooled until they can be handled, peeled, cubed, and mashed with either the back of a spoon or a potato masher.

These cakes, savory and easy to make, are especially nice in the winter both for their color and their delicious taste.

2 small serrano chilies, seeded and finely minced

2 teaspoons finely minced fresh ginger

2 teaspoons finely minced garlic

3 teaspoons chopped fresh cilantro leaves

½ teaspoon ground turmeric

½ teaspoon good-quality curry powder

Salt substitute to taste, optional

2 teaspoons fresh lime or lemon juice

3 medium sweet potatoes, baked and mashed (about 1½ to 1¾ cups)

2 tablespoons rice flour

2 tablespoons whole wheat flour

7 to 8 tablespoons cool water

Nonstick cooking spray for browning

In a small bowl, combine the chilies, ginger, garlic, cilantro, turmeric, curry powder, salt substitute, if desired, and lime juice and add this mixture to the sweet potatoes.

Mix together very thoroughly, being sure to combine all of the ingredients. Shape the mixture into small balls about 2 inches in diameter and then flatten to make small patties.

In a small bowl or a cup, combine the rice flour and whole wheat flour and whisking all the while, gradually add the cool water, 2 or 3 tablespoons at a time, until you get a very thin batter.

Heat a large, heavy-bottomed skillet or griddle over medium-high heat and lightly coat with the nonstick cooking spray. Dip the potato patties in the batter and brown in the skillet until golden and crisp. You may hold the fritters in a prewarmed 200°F oven to keep them warm while browning the others or heat them in the microwave just before serving.

YIELD: 8 fritters   SERVING SIZE: 1 fritter

Calories	Protein	Carbohydrates	Fat	Sodium
58	1 g	14 g	0 g	0 mg

Exchange: 1 starch

Rice and Pasta

Lime Rice

Herbal Baked Rice with Pine Nuts

Rice and Cranberry Stuffing

Risotto with Spinach

Fresh Corn and Wild Rice Sauté

Wild Rice and Shrimp Creole

Sautéed Acini

Bow Tie Pasta with Roasted Red, Yellow,
and Green Bell Peppers

Linguini with Clams

Spicy Chilled Soba Noodles

Lime Rice

1½ cups Chicken Broth (page 133), Vegetable Broth (page 128), low-fat, low-sodium canned broth, or water
1 cup long-grain white rice
1 tablespoon extra-virgin olive oil
2½ tablespoons fresh lime or lemon juice and 3 teaspoons grated zest (for garnish)
1 teaspoon ground white pepper
¼ cup chopped green onions or scallions for garnish

Preheat the oven to 350°F.

In a medium (2-quart) saucepan, heat the broth. Set the lime zest aside to use for garnish.

To the heated broth, add the rice, oil, lime juice, and white pepper. Pour the entire mixture into an ovenproof casserole and bake for about 1 hour. Garnish with the reserved lime zest and green onions.

YIELD: 6 servings   SERVING SIZE: ½ cup

Calories	Protein	Carbohydrates	Fat	Sodium
117	2 g	21 g	2.14 g	2.57 mg

Exchange: 1½ starches

Herbal Baked Rice with Pine Nuts

So often rice is boiled or simmered on top of the stove when it could easily be baked in the oven. Baking ensures perfectly done rice for those who have difficulty getting the consistency they want and frees up the stovetop for other cooking.

The recipe calls for toasted pine nuts. I always toast them in advance so that I will have them on hand when I need them. The easiest way to toast pine nuts is to put them in a dry skillet over medium heat and toss them until they turn golden brown, about 1 to 2 minutes. This process does not take long and greatly enhances the flavor of the nut. Both toasted and untoasted nuts will stay fresh for the same amount of time. To store them for 2 weeks or less, seal them in an airtight container and put them on a shelf. If storing them for longer, refrigerate.

1 tablespoon canola oil

3 tablespoons finely minced shallots or yellow or white onion

1½ tablespoons minced garlic

¾ cup basmati rice

1½ cups Chicken Broth (page 133), Garlic Broth (page 132), Vegetable Broth (page 128), or low-fat, low-sodium canned broth

2 large sprigs of fresh parsley, or 1 tablespoon dried, crumbled

1 large sprig of fresh tarragon, thyme, basil, or oregano, or ½ teaspoon dried, crumbled

2 small bay leaves

Dash of cayenne pepper

1 teaspoon extra-virgin olive oil

3 tablespoons toasted pine nuts

Preheat the oven to 400°F.

In a medium (2-quart) ovenproof saucepan with a tight-fitting lid, heat the canola oil over low heat. Add the shallots and garlic, and sauté, stirring gently with a spoon, until the shallots are translucent.

Add the rice and stir briefly over low heat until all of the grains are coated with the oil. Pour in the broth, stirring carefully to make sure that there are no lumps in the rice. Add the parsley, tarragon, bay leaves, and cayenne pepper, stirring to combine.

Cover the pot and place it in the oven. Bake the rice for 20 to 24 minutes (until all the liquid is absorbed).

When the rice is done, remove the parsley, tarragon, and bay leaves and using a large meat or salad fork, stir in the olive oil and pine nuts.

Either serve immediately or cover and keep warm until you are ready to eat.

YIELD: 4 servings   SERVING SIZE: ½ cup

Calories	Protein	Carbohydrates	Fat	Sodium
162	2.75 g	19.25 g	8.9 g	5.25 mg

Exchange: 1 starch; 1½ fats

Rice and Cranberry Stuffing

The rice for this dish can be cooked in advance.

½ cup wild rice or brown rice

1 cup basmati rice

3 cups Vegetable Broth (page 128), Chicken Broth (page 133), or low-fat, low-sodium canned broth

1½ tablespoons extra-virgin olive oil

1 cup chopped mushrooms

1 small yellow onion, finely diced

½ cup finely diced celery

¼ cup finely minced fresh parsley

¼ cup minced garlic

1½ tablespoons poultry seasoning

Coarsely ground black pepper to taste

½ pound fresh cranberries

If using wild rice, cook it in 1 cup of the broth for 20 to 25 minutes, until all the broth is absorbed. Cook the basmati rice separately in the remaining 2 cups of broth for about 25 minutes, or until all the broth is absorbed. If using brown rice, combine the brown rice with the basmati rice and cook the 1½ cups of rice together with the 3 cups of broth for 30 minutes, or until all the broth is absorbed.

While the rice is cooking, heat the oil in a large sauté pan and add the mushrooms, onion, celery, parsley, garlic, poultry seasoning, and pepper. Sauté until the vegetables are soft. Stir the seasoned vegetables and the cranberries into the cooked rice.

Preheat the oven to 350°F.

Put the rice mixture in an 8- or 9-inch square baking dish, cover, and bake until thoroughly heated (about 20 to 25 minutes). Serve.

Calories	Protein	Carbohydrates	Fat	Sodium
108	2.08 g	20.25 g	1.96 g	6 mg

Exchange: 1 starch; 1 vegetable

Risotto with Spinach

3½ cups Chicken Broth (page 133),
    Garlic Broth (page 132),
    Vegetable Broth (page 128), or
    low-fat, low-sodium canned broth
1 tablespoon extra-virgin olive oil
½ small yellow or white onion,
    minced
½ cup arborio or other medium-
    grain rice
¼ cup dry sherry or dry white wine
¼ cup finely grated Parmesan
    cheese

1 cup blanched chopped, fresh
    spinach, or 1 (10-ounce) package
    frozen spinach, thawed
¼ cup finely sliced fresh basil or
    chopped tarragon or marjoram
2 tablespoons fresh lime or lemon
    juice
¼ cup blanched diced red bell pepper
    for garnish, optional

Heat the broth in a medium (1½-quart) saucepan and hold at a simmer until ready to use.

Heat half of the oil in a large sauté pan over medium heat. Cook the onion for 5 to 6 minutes, until translucent. Do not brown.

Add the rice and stir, cooking for several minutes. Add the sherry and boil until it is absorbed. Add 1 cup of the simmering broth and cook, uncovered, stirring occasionally, until it is almost completely absorbed, about 7 to 8 minutes. Add the remaining broth, 6 ounces at a time, stirring occasionally, until the broth is absorbed. The total cooking time will be about 25 minutes. The risotto will be creamy, not fluffy.

Add the remaining oil, the Parmesan, spinach, basil, and lime juice, heat, and stir. Serve and sprinkle with the bell pepper, if desired.

YIELD: 4 servings   SERVING SIZE: ½ cup

Calories	Protein	Carbohydrates	Fat	Sodium
125	3 g	15 g	5 g	85 mg

Exchange: 1 starch; 1 fat

Fresh Corn and Wild Rice Sauté

The rice for this side dish needs to be cooked in advance. It can easily be cooked the day before. This works well with frozen corn kernels, but the fresh is definitely better, preferably sweet, white corn (see instructions, page 218, for cutting corn from the cob).

1 tablespoon extra-virgin olive oil

1 tablespoon canola oil

4 teaspoons minced garlic

¼ cup diced yellow onion

2 cups (about 4 medium ears) fresh or thawed frozen corn kernels

1 cup cooked wild rice or wild rice mix

3 tablespoons finely minced sun-dried tomatoes (see headnote and Note, pages 163–64)

3 tablespoons sliced fresh basil plus additional whole leaves for garnish, optional, or 2 teaspoons dried, crumbled

Salt substitute to taste

Coarsely ground black pepper to taste

1 tablespoon fresh lime or lemon juice

In a large skillet over medium heat, heat the oils. Add the garlic and sauté for about 30 seconds. Add the onion and cook for 3 to 4 minutes. Stir in the corn, wild rice, and sun-dried tomatoes and cook for 5 to 7 minutes.

Add the 3 tablespoons of sliced basil, salt substitute, and pepper. Add the lime juice, stir, and garnish with the whole basil leaves, if desired. Serve.

YIELD: 6 servings   SERVING SIZE: ½ cup

Calories	Protein	Carbohydrates	Fat	Sodium
133	3 g	22.33 g	4.33 g	10.46 mg

Exchange: 1½ starches; 1 fat

Wild Rice and Shrimp Creole

This stew is surprisingly quick and easy to make. Wild rice is one of my favorite starches. It is not a rice, but an aquatic grass, and is the only grain native to North America.

When I make this dish, I use medium shrimp, 31 to 36 shrimp to the pound, and serve the creole on a small mound of cooked white rice.

1 medium yellow onion, finely
    diced
1 small red or green bell pepper,
    stemmed, seeded, and finely diced
1 large celery stalk, finely diced
2 tablespoons unsalted, low-fat
    margarine
1 (29-ounce) can low-sodium whole
    peeled plum tomatoes, chopped,
    with their juice

1¾ cups water
½ teaspoon salt substitute
½ teaspoon cayenne pepper
1 teaspoon minced fresh garlic or
    granulated garlic
¼ teaspoon dried rosemary,
    crumbled
¼ teaspoon dried thyme,
    crumbled
1 large bay leaf, crumbled

1 (6-ounce) package long-grain and
   wild rice mix, seasoning packet
   discarded (see Note)
¾ pound shrimp, peeled,
   deveined, rinsed, and tails
   removed

1 to 1½ cups cooked white rice,
   optional
½ cup sliced green onions or
   scallions (green parts only) for
   garnish
Hot pepper sauce to taste, optional

In a medium (3-quart) saucepan, cook the yellow onion, bell pepper, and celery in the margarine for about 5 minutes or until tender.

Add the tomatoes and their juice, water, salt substitute, cayenne pepper, garlic, rosemary, thyme, and bay leaf. Stir in the rice and cover the pot. Simmer over low heat for about 20 minutes.

Add the shrimp, cover, and simmer for 10 minutes more.

If you wish, serve over a mound of warm white rice. Garnish with the green onions and pass the hot pepper sauce, if desired.

NOTE: You can also make this with long-grain white rice and wild rice that have not been commercially packaged together. Use ¼ cup of each type of rice and precook them together in the 1¾ cups of water for 20 minutes. Add the partially cooked rices and their water to the tomatoes and vegetables and proceed as above. This precooking is required because the packaged mixed rice has already been partially processed.

YIELD: 4 to 6 servings

SERVING SIZE: ⅔ cup stew plus ¼ cup rice

Calories	Protein	Carbohydrates	Fat	Sodium
150	13 g	15.5 g	3 g	154 mg

Exchange: 1 starch; 1½ lean meats

Sautéed Acini

Acini is a small pasta used in soup. It is much like barley. If it is not easily available, substitute orzo or any small round macaroni. Be sure that the acini is cooked in advance and that the other ingredients are chopped and measured ahead of time, as this dish is assembled very quickly and needs to be cooked just before serving the meal.

This dish is delicious with poultry or fish.

1 cup acini
1 tablespoon extra-virgin olive oil
2 large garlic cloves, finely minced
Salt substitute to taste, optional
1 teaspoon ground white pepper
¼ teaspoon ground nutmeg
¾ cup sliced mushrooms

⅓ cup thinly sliced green onions or scallions
1 tablespoon dry white wine, optional
2 teaspoons finely minced fresh parsley

Cook the acini until al dente, about 5 minutes, in rapidly boiling water; drain, rinse immediately in cold water, and drain again.

Heat the oil in a large, heavy-bottomed skillet over medium heat and add the acini. Season with the garlic, salt substitute, if desired, white pepper, and nutmeg. Add the mushrooms, green onions, and white wine, if desired. Move the skillet constantly over the heat until the vegetables are softened and the mixture is heated. Sprinkle the parsley over all and serve.

YIELD: **4 servings**   SERVING SIZE: **⅔ cup**

Calories	Protein	Carbohydrates	Fat	Sodium
100	2.94 g	17.3 g	3.25 g	2.3 mg

Exchange: 1 starch

Bow Tie Pasta with Roasted Red, Yellow, and Green Bell Peppers

This dish can be served hot or can be chilled in the refrigerator for several hours and served cold. See page 264 for directions on roasting the peppers.

6 medium bell peppers (2 red, 2 yellow, and 2 green), roasted, peeled, seeded, and coarsely chopped

4 green onions or scallions, thinly sliced

2 tablespoons extra-virgin olive oil

2 large garlic cloves, minced

½ teaspoon salt substitute

Coarsely ground black pepper to taste

2 cups dried bow tie pasta

2 cups broccoli florets

⅓ cup grated reduced-fat, low-sodium Parmesan cheese

2 tablespoons minced fresh parsley

¼ cup julienned fresh basil

In a large bowl, combine the bell peppers, green onions, oil, garlic, salt substitute, and pepper and set aside.

To prepare the pasta, add it to 4 quarts of rapidly boiling water and cook 7 to 8 minutes, until just tender. Drain and return the pasta to the large pot in which it was cooked.

Meanwhile, plunge the broccoli florets into boiling water for 1 minute and then immediately remove them from the water, drain, and set aside.

In the large pot, toss the pasta, roasted pepper mixture, broccoli, Parmesan cheese, and parsley.

Serve immediately or chill the dish for about 2 hours. Garnish with the basil.

YIELD: 4 servings   SERVING SIZE: ⅔ cup

Calories	Protein	Carbohydrates	Fat	Sodium
278	11 g	34 g	8.88 g	123 mg

Exchange: 2 starches; 1 lean meat; 1 fat

Linguini with Clams

This dish is usually served as an entrée with a salad. You may use any straight, thin pasta, such as linguini, fettuccine, spaghetti, or angel hair. I prefer fresh pasta over dried pasta, as it has better flavor and is faster to cook.

The cooking time for the clam sauce is about 4 minutes, so it is a good idea to have the ingredients already prepared and measured. If dried pasta is used, have it cooked, warm, and ready to go. If using fresh pasta, cook it at the same time as you cook the clam sauce.

1 pound fresh linguini, or 4 ounces dried

1 tablespoon extra-virgin olive oil

3/4 pound shelled fresh or low-sodium canned clams, chopped

1/2 cup Chicken Broth (page 133) or low-fat, low-sodium canned broth

1/4 cup dry white wine

1 (8-ounce) bottle low-sodium clam juice or clam nectar

3 tablespoons minced garlic

3 tablespoons minced shallots or onion

1/2 large red bell pepper, cut into small dice

Salt substitute to taste

Coarsely ground black pepper to taste

2 tablespoons minced fresh parsley for garnish

If using fresh pasta, bring a large pot of water to a boil and cook the pasta now until al dente, about 2 minutes. Drain and keep warm. If using dried pasta, cook according to package directions and keep warm until the sauce is done.

Heat a skillet over medium heat and add half of the oil. When the oil is hot, add the clams and quickly add the chicken broth, white wine, and clam juice. Immediately add the garlic and shallots.

Simmer for about 2 minutes, and then add the bell pepper, salt substitute, and black pepper and cook for about 1 minute more. Stir in the remaining olive oil.

Toss the clam sauce with the cooked pasta. Turn into a bowl, garnish with the parsley, and serve.

YIELD: 6 servings   SERVING SIZE: ½ cup

Calories	Protein	Carbohydrates	Fat	Sodium
132	10 g	16 g	3.33 g	115 mg

Exchange: 1 starch; ½ lean meat; ½ fat

Spicy Chilled Soba Noodles

These chilled noodles may easily be used as a snack as well as a vegetable side dish.

Soba noodles are Japanese noodles made from buckwheat flour. They are available at every Asian market, carried at many health food stores, and sold at many large supermarkets. They are very versatile and delicious whether served hot, at room temperature, or cold. Soba noodles work equally well in side dishes and salads and have more flavor than most pastas do. They can be cooked a few hours beforehand but should be carefully wrapped and refrigerated to keep them from drying out.

This dish requires chilling for several hours before serving.

Dash of salt substitute
1 pound Japanese soba noodles
½ large red bell pepper, julienned
3 large celery stalks, sliced on the diagonal
5 green onions or scallions, sliced on the diagonal
½ cup drained sliced low-sodium canned water chestnuts
1 tablespoon canola oil
½ teaspoon sesame oil

1½ tablespoons balsamic or aged red wine vinegar
3 tablespoons low-sodium soy sauce
3 tablespoons granulated sugar substitute
1½ to 2½ tablespoons Vietnamese chili paste (very, very hot), mashed fresh red chilies, Sambal Oeleck (see headnote, page 207), or Tabasco, to taste
½ large bunch of fresh cilantro leaves, chopped

Bring 4 quarts of water and the salt substitute to a boil in a large pot over medium-high heat. Soba noodles usually are packaged in 4 small bundles. Break each bundle in half and drop the noodles into the rapidly boiling water. Cook no more than 1 or 2 minutes, depending on the thickness of the noodles. With chopsticks or a spaghetti turner, lift and separate the noodles to prevent them from clumping. After you have cooked the noodles for 1 minute, check so that you will know when they are al dente.

Immediately remove the pan from the heat, drain the noodles, and rinse them under cold running water to rid them of excess starch. Drain well.

Toss the noodles in a large bowl with the bell pepper, celery, green onions, and water chestnuts.

Combine the oils, vinegar, soy sauce, sugar substitute, and chili paste. Pour the dressing over the noodle mixture and toss until evenly coated. Chill.

When you are ready to serve, add the cilantro and toss.

YIELD: 8 servings   SERVING SIZE: ½ cup

Calories	Protein	Carbohydrates	Fat	Sodium
212	8 g	43 g	2.34 g	297.31 mg

Exchange: 2½ starches

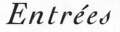

Entrées

About Marinating

Roasting Peppers

Lime Chicken Breasts

Roasted Chicken Breasts

Greek Chicken

Broiled Chicken Tarragon with Wine

Spiced Chicken with Spinach

Grilled or Broiled Chicken with
Vegetable Vinaigrette

Chicken Provençale

Tofu Chicken Casserole with Mushrooms
and Artichokes

Honeyed Chicken Breasts

Red Pepper Steak

Poached Salmon

Spiced Baked Fish

Steamed or Microwaved Ginger Fish with Soy

Broiled Fish with Tomatoes, Garlic, and Chilies

Baked Flounder with Ginger and Oranges

Grilled or Broiled Tuna with
Mango-Papaya Relish

Braised Salmon and Halibut Steaks

Stir-fried Shrimp with Peas and
Water Chestnuts

Halibut Kebabs

Portuguese Fish Stew

Ceviche

Tofu-and-Cheese-Stuffed Jumbo Shells

Baked Chiles Rellenos

About Marinating

The French word *marinade* comes from the Italian *marinare*, meaning to soak in a piquant liquid prior to cooking. The liquid can consist of wine, cider, or an acid such as vinegar or lime juice, which is then flavored with herbs, spices, and onions, and is often enriched with oil. Some Asian and Eastern European marinades contain yogurt. The marinade mixture is frequently strained and used as a base for a sauce to accompany the food that was marinated.

We choose the marinating process for two reasons: for the enhanced flavor it adds as well as for what it can do for the texture of the food.

When you marinate chicken, pork, tofu, or even vegetables, you are able to add flavor to these foods. This technique can give something relatively bland a sharp, well-rounded flavor. It can also mellow out a strong, perhaps undesirable, flavor. The enhanced flavor comes from the herbs, spices, and/or onions that the marinade contains. The strength of the ingredients and the length of time the food rests in the marinade affect the intensity of the flavor.

Oil is added to a marinade to provide moisture and keep the food from sticking to cooking surfaces. Olive oil or canola oil is the best choice.

Marinating can also tenderize tough cuts of meat or poultry and break down stringy meats. If you let fish rest long enough in a marinade, with enough citrus, the acid in the marinade, be it vinegar, citrus juice, wine, or tomato products, will literally "cook" the fish.

Always marinate items in the refrigerator unless you are really pressed for time. In a pinch you can marinate at room temperature for 1 or 2 hours. Turn the food every hour or so, so that all sides have contact with the liquid. Use an acid-resistant container such as stainless steel, glass, nonporous ceramic, or plastic so that the acid in the marinade does not interact with the vessel.

Roasting Peppers

To roast peppers in the oven or broiler, preheat the oven to 500°F. Place the peppers on a sheet pan or cookie sheet and cook until the skins start to wrinkle or turn brown. Periodically rotate the peppers so that they are uniformly cooked. Remove the peppers from the pan, let cool, and then peel and seed them.

I prefer to roast peppers by searing them on top of the stove. This can be done only with a gas stove, as the procedure is done directly over the flame. Either hold the peppers over the flame with a pair of tongs or lay the peppers directly on top of the burner. The second method is my favorite, as it enables me to do more than one at a time. Rotate the peppers with tongs until all the sides, tops, and bottoms are blackened. Many people then put the blackened peppers in a plastic or paper bag and allow them to steam for 10 minutes or so before peeling and seeding them. I plunge them immediately into a big bowl of ice and water to stop the cooking. This procedure leaves them crisp and sets their color. Both roasting methods give you peppers that are easy to seed and peel.

Roasted peppers can be stored in oil and vinegar with garlic, and if refrigerated, can be stored for about 6 weeks.

Lime Chicken Breasts

This dish requires at least 1 hour for the chicken to marinate and can be held in the refrigerator for up to 10 hours (see About Marinating, page 263). Red and yellow bell peppers taste delicious and make the presentation something special. In the interest of economy, however, green bell peppers can be substituted.

4 (4- to 5-ounce) boneless, skinless chicken breasts, trimmed of excess fat

2 tablespoons extra-virgin olive oil

Grated zest and juice of 2 medium limes or lemons

3 large garlic cloves, minced

1 small yellow onion, diced

Pinch of salt, optional

Coarsely ground black pepper to taste

5 tablespoons finely chopped fresh cilantro leaves

2 medium bell peppers

Cut out the chicken tenderloin from the underside of each breast. The tenderloin is that elongated, boneless flap of meat on the underside of the breast that is fairly thin and runs from top to bottom. The tenderloins may be used in this recipe, in which case an extra person can easily be fed, or you may freeze the tenders for future use.

Flatten the breasts and tenders, if you are using them, with a meat mallet (a mallet, often wooden, that has a square head with pointed nubs for pounding out meats) between sheets of waxed paper or plastic wrap. If you do not have a meat mallet, you can roll out the breasts with a rolling pin or a bottle. Place the flattened breasts in a nonreactive dish large enough to hold the marinade.

In a small bowl, combine the oil, lime zest and juice, garlic, onion, salt, if desired, and pepper, and 2 tablespoons of the cilantro and pour it over the chicken to marinate for 1 hour.

Meanwhile, roast, peel, seed, and julienne the peppers (see Roasting Peppers, page 264).

Remove the breasts from the marinade and grill over medium-hot coals or broil under medium heat for about 2 minutes on each side. Remove the breasts from the grill or broiler and put on a platter or individual plates. Sprinkle the remaining cilantro over the breasts and serve with the roasted peppers.

YIELD: 4 servings   SERVING SIZE: 1 breast

Calories	Protein	Carbohydrates	Fat	Sodium
204	27 g	1 g	9.5 g	64 mg

Exchange: 3 lean meats; 1 fat

Roasted Chicken Breasts

Marinate the chicken for at least 45 minutes in the refrigerator; the flavor will be best when the chicken is in the marinade for several hours. You can do it in the morning to cook in the evening, but you should not leave chicken in a marinade for any longer than 8 hours — it will get spongy.

3 medium garlic cloves, minced

1 heaping tablespoon minced fresh
   ginger, or 1½ teaspoons ground

2 teaspoons ground coriander

1 teaspoon ground white pepper

½ teaspoon salt substitute, optional

1 tablespoon canola oil

4 (4- to 5-ounce) boneless, skinless
   chicken breasts, trimmed of
   excess fat

In a small bowl, combine the garlic, ginger, coriander, white pepper, and salt substitute, if desired. Add the oil and after mixing thoroughly, rub the marinade on the chicken. Refrigerate in a non-reactive dish for at least 45 minutes.

Preheat the oven to 350°F.

Bake the breasts, uncovered, for 20 to 25 minutes. Serve with Cabbage Salad (page 185).

YIELD: 4 servings   SERVING SIZE: 1 breast

Calories	Protein	Carbohydrates	Fat	Sodium
171	27 g	0 g	6.5 g	64 mg

Exchange: 4 lean meats

Greek Chicken

¼ cup all-purpose unbleached flour
⅛ teaspoon paprika
⅛ teaspoon finely ground black
    pepper
4 (4- to 5-ounce) boneless, skinless
    chicken breasts, trimmed of
    excess fat
Nonstick cooking spray for
    sautéing
3 small shallots, minced
¾ cup sliced mushrooms
3 large garlic cloves, minced

1 teaspoon minced fresh parsley
1 teaspoon dried oregano
¼ cup dry white wine
½ cup Chicken Broth (page 133),
    Garlic Broth (page 132),
    Vegetable Broth (page 128), or
    low-fat, low-sodium canned broth
2 tablespoons crumbled feta cheese
¾ cup diced ripe plum tomatoes
½ cup thinly sliced green onions or
    scallions
Thinly sliced fresh basil for garnish

Preheat the oven to 250°F.

Season the flour with the paprika and pepper. Dredge the chicken breasts in the seasoned flour, shaking off the excess flour. Heat a large, heavy-bottomed skillet over medium-high heat, lightly coat it with the nonstick cooking spray, and sauté the breasts on both sides until they are golden brown.

Remove the chicken from the skillet and hold in the oven while you prepare the sauce.

To the sauté skillet, add the shallots, mushrooms, garlic, parsley, and oregano. Sauté lightly over medium heat for 3 to 4 minutes and then add the white wine, all the while moving the pan rapidly.

Add the broth and feta cheese, whisking to blend the cheese. Add the tomato, stir, and place the chicken breasts back in the skillet. Stir in the green onions. Cook for 2 to 3 minutes. Remove the breasts from the skillet, spoon the sauce over them, and garnish with the basil.

YIELD: 4 servings   SERVING SIZE: 1 breast

Calories	Protein	Carbohydrates	Fat	Sodium
213	29 g	7.44 g	6.06 g	146.94 mg

Exchange: 4 lean meats; ½ starch

Broiled Chicken Tarragon with Wine

This marinade uses a good bit of wine, so ask a knowledgeable person at the wine shop to help you purchase wine with a low sodium content.

The chicken breasts should rest in the marinade in the refrigerator for about 1 hour before broiling.

⅓ cup fresh tarragon, or 2½ tablespoons dried
5 shallots, finely minced
2 large garlic cloves, minced
1¼ cups dry white wine

4 (4- to 5-ounce) boneless, skinless chicken breasts, trimmed of excess fat
1 tablespoon extra-virgin olive oil
Curly endive or kale leaves for garnish, optional

In a small bowl, combine the tarragon, shallots, garlic, and white wine. Rub the chicken breasts with the oil. Place the breasts in a nonreactive dish large enough to hold the marinade and pour the marinade over them. Cover and refrigerate for about 1 hour.

Preheat the broiler.

Remove the breasts from the marinade, place on the broiler pan, and put under the broiler. Strain the marinade and while the breasts are broiling, baste them at least once on each side to keep them moist. Save the marinade you have left over. Each side should be cooked for 5 to 6 minutes, at which point the breasts should be tender.

Remove the chicken and keep it warm on a serving platter or individual plates, leaving any marinade and tidbits in the bottom of the broiler pan.

Place the broiler pan on top of the stove and pour the reserved marinade in the pan. Heat while scraping the pan with a spatula or wooden spoon to remove all of the tidbits from the pan. Pour the juices on the chicken, garnish with the endive, if desired, and serve.

YIELD: 4 servings   SERVING SIZE: 1 breast

Calories	Protein	Carbohydrates	Fat	Sodium
233	27.25 g	2.75 g	6.5 g	68 mg

Exchange: 4 lean meats

Spiced Chicken with Spinach

If you buy a whole chicken and cut it up yourself, you will have parts you do not use (the back, the neck, etc.) to wrap and freeze until you have enough to make Chicken Broth (page 133), and you will pay less per pound than if you bought chicken parts.

1 (2½- to 3-pound) chicken, cut into 8 pieces, skinned, and trimmed of excess fat

All-purpose flour for dusting the chicken

1½ to 2 tablespoons canola oil

2 small yellow onions, finely diced

2 ripe medium tomatoes, or 1 (8-ounce) can low-sodium whole peeled plum tomatoes, drained and chopped

2 small bunches of fresh spinach (about 1 pound), thoroughly washed, stemmed, drained, and coarsely chopped

3 medium garlic cloves, minced

1 teaspoon ground coriander

Coarsely ground black pepper to taste

3 whole cloves

¼ teaspoon ground turmeric

¼ teaspoon good-quality curry powder

Salt to taste, optional

¼ cup skim milk

Dust the chicken with the flour and using about half of the oil, lightly brown on both sides in a large skillet over medium heat. After the chicken is browned, remove from the skillet and set aside.

Preheat the oven to 350°F.

In the same skillet over medium heat, heat the rest of the oil and cook the onions for about 5 minutes. Add the tomatoes, spinach, garlic, spices, and salt, if desired, and cook for 5 minutes more. Add the milk and mix well.

Place the vegetable mixture in a 3- or 4-quart ovenproof casserole dish, arrange the chicken pieces on top, cover tightly, and bake until the chicken is tender, 40 to 45 minutes. Serve.

YIELD: 4 servings   SERVING SIZE: 2 pieces of chicken

Calories	Protein	Carbohydrates	Fat	Sodium
244	27 g	8.1 g	9.38 g	161 mg

Exchange: 3 lean meats; 1½ vegetables

Grilled or Broiled Chicken with Vegetable Vinaigrette

Jicama is a root vegetable about the size of a small potato and with a similar brown, rough skin. It is slightly sweet in flavor and very crisp. It adds a nice texture and flavor to any dish. It is native to Mexico, California, and the Southwest.

The chicken breasts should be marinated for at least 1½ hours. They can be put in the marinade late in the morning for cooking that evening.

4 (4- to 5-ounce) boneless, skinless
   chicken breasts, trimmed of
   excess fat
1 cup homemade vinaigrette or low-
   calorie, low-fat commercial
   vinaigrette
2 small red bell peppers, stemmed
   and seeded

2 small zucchini
2 small yellow crookneck
   squash
2 medium carrots, peeled
1 small jicama
8 fresh or thawed frozen asparagus
   spears

Place the chicken breasts in a glass or stainless steel bowl and cover them with ½ cup of the vinaigrette. Refrigerate for at least 1½ hours.

Cut the vegetables into ¼-inch-wide strips and put into the remainder of the vinaigrette, tossing gently to coat. Cover and hold the vegetables on the side until ready to cook. It is not necessary to refrigerate, unless you are preparing them in advance.

Have boiling water ready in a medium pan with a steamer insert to steam the vegetables.

Remove the chicken from the marinade, saving the marinade. Grill the chicken over medium-hot coals for 3 to 4 minutes on each side, or broil under medium heat for about the same amount of time. Baste the chicken with the marinade at least twice during the cooking, once on each side. Discard the chicken marinade after you have finished basting the chicken.

Remove the vegetables from the marinade and steam them, covered, for 3 to 4 minutes. The vegetables should be tender-crisp.

Divide the vegetables among 4 plates and serve the chicken on top. You may wish to drizzle the remainder of the marinade from the vegetables over the entrée. Serve.

YIELD: 4 servings   SERVING SIZE: 1 breast

Calories	Protein	Carbohydrates	Fat	Sodium
201	30 g	14 g	3.5 g	216.5 mg

Exchange: 4 lean meats; 2 vegetables

Chicken Provençale

1 (14½-ounce) can low-sodium whole peeled plum tomatoes, chopped, with their juice

3 tablespoons pitted and sliced ripe olives

1 tablespoon minced fresh basil, or 3 teaspoons dried, crumbled

4 medium garlic cloves, minced

1 egg white, beaten

2 teaspoons water

⅓ cup fine dry bread crumbs (see Note)

3 tablespoons minced fresh parsley

Coarsely ground black pepper to taste

4 (4- to 5-ounce) boneless, skinless chicken breasts, trimmed of excess fat

2 teaspoons extra-virgin olive oil

4 ounces dried fettuccine or linguini or 8 ounces fresh

1 large carrot, peeled and sliced into long julienne

1 large zucchini, peeled and sliced lengthwise into ½-inch-wide strips

1 tablespoon low-fat, low-sodium margarine

Grated Parmesan cheese to taste, optional

In a small saucepan, combine the tomatoes, olives, basil, and garlic and let sit until needed.

In a small bowl, whisk together the egg white and the water. In a pie pan or a shallow dish, mix the bread crumbs, parsley, and pepper. After rinsing the breasts and patting them dry, dip them in the egg mixture and roll them in the seasoned bread crumbs.

Preheat the oven to 350°F.

In a large sauté pan, heat the oil and lightly sauté the breasts until they are golden. After both sides have been browned, place the breasts in the oven in a pie pan and cook until done, about 15 minutes.

Meanwhile, bring a pot of water to boil for the pasta. Heat the tomato mixture over medium heat, uncovered, for 8 to 9 minutes. Keep it warm for serving.

Cook the fettuccine for 7 to 8 minutes if it is dried or 3 to 4 minutes if it is fresh. During the last minute or so of the cooking, add the carrot and zucchini and then drain the pasta mixture and gently toss with the margarine.

Divide the pasta among four plates, serve the chicken breasts on top, and pour ½ cup of sauce over each breast. Sprinkle with the Parmesan cheese, if desired.

N O T E : To make bread crumbs, take whatever old bread or rolls you have on hand. Put them on a cookie sheet and toast them in a 350°F oven until the bread is golden brown and hard through and through. This can also be done in a toaster oven, but the bread does require more watching than if you cook it in the oven. Break the bread into small chunks and place in the bowl of a food processor. Using the steel blade, process the bread until it is in crumbs. The length of time you process depends on the kind of crumbs you want — fine, coarse, etc.

If you want seasoned bread crumbs, mix in minced parsley, grated Parmesan, and granulated garlic. You need never buy bread crumbs again and you will not have to throw out any old bread or rolls. Just put the bread crumbs in a plastic bag and freeze.

YIELD: 4 servings

SERVING SIZE: 1 breast, scant ⅔ cup pasta and vegetables, and ½ cup of sauce

Calories	Protein	Carbohydrates	Fat	Sodium
245	30 g	12 g	8.72 g	288 mg

Exchange: 3 lean meats; 1 starch

Tofu Chicken Casserole with Mushrooms and Artichokes

This casserole is simple to make, and the taste is fabulous. For the diabetic, it's like the best of both worlds: plenty of flavor, very little animal protein, and very little fat. For the cook, it's something that can be put together quickly that everyone will enjoy and that is tasty enough to serve for company or for any special occasion. I usually use chicken breasts for this dish, but any boneless, skinless piece of chicken will do nicely.

Nonstick cooking spray for the
   baking dish and sautéing
1 pound extra-firm tofu
¾ pound boneless, skinless chicken
   breasts or thighs, trimmed of
   excess fat
2 cups sliced mushrooms
1 cup Chicken Broth (page 133),
   Garlic Broth (page 132),
   Vegetable Broth (page 128), or
   low-fat, low-sodium canned
   broth

2 tablespoons cornstarch dissolved
   in ¼ cup cold water
2 tablespoons plain nonfat yogurt
1 tablespoon dry sherry
½ teaspoon salt substitute
Coarsely ground black pepper to
   taste
1 teaspoon dried tarragon
1 teaspoon garlic powder
1 cup halved fresh or thawed frozen
   artichoke hearts
Dash of paprika

Preheat the oven to 375°F.

Lightly coat a 2- or 3-quart ovenproof casserole with the nonstick cooking spray and set aside.

Drain the block of tofu and press it between several thicknesses of paper towels to remove the excess moisture. Cut the tofu into ½-inch slices. You should have about 1⅔ cups. Heat a medium skillet, lightly coat it with the nonstick cooking spray, and when it is hot, brown the pieces of tofu until they are golden brown, drain, and set aside.

Heat the same skillet again and apply more nonstick cooking spray if necessary. Lightly brown the chicken on both sides, drain, pull the chicken into smaller pieces, and set aside.

Heat the skillet again and if necessary reapply the nonstick cooking spray. When the skillet is hot, toss in the sliced mushrooms and lightly brown them. Remove the skillet from the heat and hold on the side.

Heat the broth in a saucepan and add the dissolved cornstarch. Add the yogurt, sherry, salt substitute, pepper, tarragon, and garlic. Cook on low heat until the sauce is warmed through and immediately turn it into the skillet with the mushrooms. Over a low heat, mix the ingredients thoroughly to pick up the flavor of the browned juices and the tidbits in the pan.

In the prepared casserole dish, layer the tofu, chicken, and the artichokes, repeating the layers until all of the ingredients are gone. Pour the sauce and the mushrooms on top. Sprinkle the paprika over the top and bake for about 40 minutes. At this point the dish should be nicely browned. Serve.

YIELD: 6 servings　　　　　SERVING SIZE: 1 cup

Calories	Protein	Carbohydrates	Fat	Sodium
165	19 g	5 g	7 g	67 mg

Exchange: 2 medium-fat meats; 1 vegetable

Honeyed Chicken Breasts

I recommend boneless, skinless breasts for this recipe, but you can use skinned chicken parts with the bone in just as easily and, if you are going to serve a large number of people, more economically. This dish requires a bit of work but is ideal for entertaining as the recipe can easily be doubled or tripled.

Some refrigeration is required after the initial cooking, which can be done either the night before or the morning of the day you plan to serve it.

1 medium onion, halved lengthwise
and sliced

1 large celery stalk, sliced into
1-inch-long pieces

1 large carrot, peeled and cut into
1-inch-long pieces

3 large sprigs of fresh parsley

½ teaspoon salt substitute

½ to 1 teaspoon ground white
pepper

1 teaspoon dried thyme,
crumbled

1 large bay leaf

2 large garlic cloves, minced

1½ to 2 cups Chicken Broth (page
133) or low-fat, low-sodium
canned broth

1 cup water

6 (4- to 5-ounce) boneless, skinless
chicken breasts, trimmed of
excess fat

¼ cup sliced almonds

⅓ cup honey

Kale leaves for garnish, optional

2 tart green apples, thinly sliced
and briefly soaked in pineapple
juice or orange juice for garnish,
optional

In a large (6-quart), heavy pot, combine the onion, celery, carrot, parsley, salt substitute, white pepper, thyme, bay leaf, garlic, broth, and water. Bring this mixture to a boil, add the chicken, and lower the heat. Simmer, covered, for 15 to 20 minutes, at which point the chicken breasts should be tender. (It will take 30 to 35 minutes cooking for other bone-in chicken parts.)

Remove the pot from the heat and let the mixture cool. At this point you can cover the pot and refrigerate, or very carefully transfer the contents to another dish, cover, and refrigerate. Refrigerate the chicken for at least 4 hours or overnight.

When you are ready to cook, remove the pot from the refrigerator and heat for 10 to 15 minutes over low heat, until the chicken is warmed through.

Preheat the broiler.

Arrange the almonds in a single layer in a pie tin. Broil for about 1 minute, stirring frequently, until they are golden brown. Watch closely, as they burn easily. Set aside.

Remove the chicken from the broth and place it, serving side down, in a large, shallow broiler pan. Strain the broth and set aside.

Broil the chicken under medium heat for about 2 minutes. When broiling, keep the chicken about 5 inches from the heat source.

Turn the pieces over. Spoon about ¾ cup of the broth over the chicken and refrigerate or freeze the rest for future use. Using a pastry brush or a designated kitchen paintbrush, paint the top (the serving side) of the chicken with about half of the honey and broil for about 3 minutes. Brush with the rest of the honey and broil until the chicken is glazed and golden brown.

Sprinkle the chicken with the toasted almonds. Remove the chicken from the broiler pan and place on a warmed platter and garnish with the kale and sliced apples, if desired.

YIELD: 6 servings   SERVING SIZE: 1 breast

Calories	Protein	Carbohydrates	Fat	Sodium
290	29 g	27 g	8 g	76 mg

Exchange: 4 lean meats; 2 vegetables; 1 fruit

Red Pepper Steak

The marinated beef can be prepared ahead of time and held in the refrigerator until you are ready to cook. I usually let it sit in the marinade for about 1 hour, but it can easily be held all day.

½ pound round steak, trimmed of excess fat (any fairly lean, inexpensive cut of steak can be used as well)

5 tablespoons reduced- or low-sodium soy sauce

1 large garlic clove, minced

2 teaspoons minced fresh ginger, or ⅔ teaspoon ground

Nonstick cooking spray for sautéing

½ cup thinly sliced red onion

½ cup thinly sliced green onions or scallions

1 large red bell pepper, stemmed, seeded, and cut into 1-inch squares (about 1 cup)

1 large celery stalk, thinly sliced

⅓ cup drained sliced low-sodium canned water chestnuts

1 tablespoon cornstarch dissolved in ½ cup cold water

2 large ripe tomatoes, cut into wedges

¼ cup chopped fresh cilantro leaves for garnish, optional

Slice the beef across the grain into very thin strips.

In a large bowl, combine the soy sauce, garlic, and ginger and add the beef. Toss the mixture and hold on the side while you prepare the vegetables.

Spray a large skillet or a wok with the cooking spray and heat over high heat. Toss in the beef and quickly brown. At this point, the meat should be tender. If not, sauté for 5 minutes more and then add the red and green onions, bell pepper, celery, and water chestnuts. Toss until the vegetables are tender-crisp, 4 to 5 minutes.

Push the beef and vegetable sauté to the side of the pan and add the dissolved cornstarch, cooking the juices until thickened. Toss the sauté with the thickened sauce until thoroughly mixed and add the tomatoes, mixing gently. Divide into servings and garnish with the cilantro, if desired.

YIELD: 4 servings   SERVING SIZE: ¾ cup

Calories	Protein	Carbohydrates	Fat	Sodium
182	15.5 g	7 g	7.26 g	860 mg

Exchange: 2 lean meats; ½ starch; ½ fat

Poached Salmon

This dish is really delicious when served with Dilled Cucumber Salad (page 193). Use a flavorful wine, such as a Chardonnay or Riesling. The alcohol will cook out, but the flavor remains.

2 cups dry white wine
1 cup water
3 large bay leaves
4 small onions
15 whole black peppercorns
1 tablespoon fresh dill, or 1 teaspoon dried, crumbled

2 garlic cloves
2 pounds salmon (preferably a side of salmon, but smaller fillets or salmon steaks may be used)

Fill a fish poacher or flat roaster or large, rather deep baking pan with all of the ingredients except the salmon and bring to a boil. Place the fish on the rack; if you are not using a poacher, wrap the fish in cheesecloth, which will keep the fish intact during cooking. Lower the heat to a simmer and poach for 8 to 10 minutes. The fish is done when a knife inserted comes out clean.

YIELD: 8 servings   SERVING SIZE: 3 ounces

Calories	Protein	Carbohydrates	Fat	Sodium
186	21.13 g	1.94 g	5 g	57.94 mg

Exchange: 3 lean meats

Spiced Baked Fish

For this dish I prefer to use red snapper. However, Pacific snapper, drum, redfish, sole, perch, orange roughy, or any firm-fleshed fillet may be used with equal success, but the fish must be very fresh.

If you are limited to frozen fish, quickly thaw it by putting it in an airtight bag and running cold water over it, or defrost it in the microwave. In either case, be sure to pat thoroughly dry with paper towels before cooking.

1 pound red snapper or firm-fleshed
    fish, cut into 4 (4-ounce) fillets
¾ cup plain nonfat yogurt
1½ tablespoons fresh lime or lemon
    juice
1½ tablespoons minced fresh ginger
3 serrano chilies, seeded and minced

3 or 4 whole cloves
Heaping ¼ teaspoon ground
    cardamom
1 teaspoon ground coriander
1 teaspoon granulated sugar
    substitute
1 tablespoon minced fresh garlic

Preheat the oven to 350°F.

Rinse the fillets, pat them dry, and place them in a 9-by-13-inch flat baking dish.

In a small bowl, combine the yogurt and lime juice and add the remaining ingredients. Whisk until well mixed and pour over the fish. Cover the fish either with a lid or with foil and bake for 25 to 30 minutes. Serve.

YIELD: 4 servings   SERVING SIZE: 3 ounces

Calories	Protein	Carbohydrates	Fat	Sodium
108	19.69 g	4.19 g	1 g	134 mg

Exchange: 3 lean meats

Steamed or Microwaved Ginger Fish with Soy

This fish is especially great to prepare and serve during the warmer months, as it is either steamed on top of the stove or cooked in the microwave and therefore does not heat up the kitchen. It is light and delicate in taste, making it a good summer entrée, but it is also great to serve during the winter months, as none of its ingredients are seasonal.

You will need either a large bamboo steamer (available at any health food store or Asian market) or a metal steamer with a basket. The small metal steamer with the pole in the middle will not work, as the fish is steamed on the plate you use to serve it, and the plate will not fit on the ordinary small vegetable steamer.

If you choose to microwave the fish, cook the fish on its serving plate. The plate prevents the fish from falling apart too easily and gives you only one dish to wash.

1 pound sea bass, trout, drum, redfish, or other firm-fleshed white fish (use either a thick fillet or a side of fish with at least a ½-inch thickness)
2 tablespoons minced fresh ginger

4 green onions or scallions (green parts only), cut into 2-inch lengths and then cut lengthwise into julienne
3 tablespoons reduced- or low-sodium soy sauce
¼ teaspoon sesame oil

Bring several inches of water to a boil in the bottom of a steamer pot. Be sure the steamer is large enough to accommodate a plate to steam the fish on. Put the steamer insert in the pot and cover.

Place the fish on a plate and sprinkle the ginger and green onions evenly over the fish.

Meanwhile, in a small bowl, whisk the soy sauce and sesame oil briskly to combine.

Place the plate of fish in the steamer and steam for 3 to 4 minutes. The fish should be flaky when done. Drizzle the soy sauce mixture over the fish and serve.

To cook in the microwave, put 2 teaspoons of water in the bottom of the plate with the seasoned raw fish, loosely wrap with plastic wrap, and microwave on high for about 4 minutes. Take the plate out of the microwave and drain off the liquid. Drizzle the soy sauce mixture over the fish and serve.

YIELD: 4 servings   SERVING SIZE: 3 ounces

Calories	Protein	Carbohydrates	Fat	Sodium
84	17 g	1 g	1 g	396 mg

Exchange: 3 lean meats

Broiled Fish with Tomatoes, Garlic, and Chilies

Unless the recipe specifies otherwise, when you broil fish, always broil the fillets 5 inches from the heat source.

1 pound red snapper, Pacific snapper, redfish, drum, or flounder, cut into 4 (4-ounce) fillets

2 ripe medium tomatoes, scalded, peeled, and chopped, or 4 canned low-sodium whole peeled plum tomatoes, chopped, with their juice

1 tablespoon minced garlic

2 small serrano chilies, or 1 medium jalapeño pepper, minced

½ small red onion, finely diced

Coarsely ground black pepper to taste

1 tablespoon extra-virgin olive oil

2 tablespoons chopped fresh cilantro leaves or thinly sliced green onions or scallions (green parts only)

Lime or lemon wedges for garnish

Preheat the broiler.

Lay the fish fillets skin side down on a broiling pan or cookie sheet. In a small bowl, combine the tomatoes, garlic, chilies, and onion with the pepper and oil and spoon over the fillets.

Broil the fish for 5 to 6 minutes, depending on the thickness of the fillets. Baste now and again with the juices as you broil. You will want the tops of the fillets lightly browned and the fish cooked through.

Garnish the fish with the cilantro and lime wedges.

YIELD: 4 servings   SERVING SIZE: 3 ounces

Calories	Protein	Carbohydrates	Fat	Sodium
136	18 g	5 g	4.5 g	107 mg

Exchange: 3 lean meats

Baked Flounder with Ginger and Oranges

Although I like to use fresh flounder with this dish, I also use black drum, sea bass, or red or Pacific snapper. You need a fish with a thick fillet, because you will be making crosswise cuts into the fillets for the flavoring juices to penetrate.

1 pound flounder, cut into 4 (4-ounce) fillets

2 oranges

1 tablespoon plus 1 teaspoon reduced- or low-sodium soy sauce

1 teaspoon canola oil

½ teaspoon ground white pepper

3 teaspoons grated fresh ginger

Preheat the oven to 375°F.

Arrange the fish in a 9-by-13-inch ovenproof baking dish and with a paring knife, lightly trace lines across the width of the fillets at about

1-inch intervals. Do the same up and down the length of the fillets, also at about 1-inch intervals.

Finely grate the zest of 1 orange to measure 2 teaspoons. Cut the orange in half and squeeze it to get 3 tablespoons of juice.

In a small bowl, combine the orange juice, soy sauce, and oil and then whisk in the white pepper, ginger, and orange zest.

Spoon the mixture over the fish, being sure to place most of the ginger and orange zest on the fillets themselves. Cover. Bake the fish for 10 to 12 minutes, depending on the thickness of the fillets. The fish should be moist in the center but look firm and white.

Cut the remaining orange into wedges for garnish. Lift the fillets from the baking pan and serve, garnishing with the orange wedges.

YIELD: 4 servings   SERVING SIZE: 3 ounces

Calories	Protein	Carbohydrates	Fat	Sodium
96	17.1 g	1.43 g	2.16 g	321 mg

Exchange: 3 lean meats

Grilled or Broiled Tuna with Mango-Papaya Relish

I like to make this relish with mango and papaya, but they are not always available; pineapple, peaches, or oranges may be substituted for one or both of the fruits. Prepare and measure the ingredients for the relish so that it can be assembled quickly.

Use either yellowfin or bluefin tuna; I prefer the yellowfin, as it has a more delicate flavor.

Mango-Papaya Relish

1 large mango, peeled, pitted, and diced, or bottled mango slices packed in water, drained

1 large papaya, peeled, seeded, and diced

1 small red onion, finely diced

2 teaspoons minced garlic

2 serrano chilies, seeded and minced

2 tablespoons fresh lime or lemon juice

¼ cup finely minced fresh cilantro leaves

1 ounce rum, optional

Grilled or Broiled Tuna

6 (4- to 5-ounce) tuna steaks, ½-inch to ¾-inch thick

1 tablespoon canola oil

Salt to taste

Ground white pepper to taste

½ teaspoon ground coriander

1 lime or lemon cut into thick wedges

To make the relish, combine the mango, papaya, onion, garlic, chilies, lime juice, cilantro, and rum, if desired. Thoroughly mix and hold on the side.

To make the tuna, heat the broiler or heat a grill to medium-hot. Brush the tuna steaks with the oil and season with the salt, white pepper, and coriander.

Grill or broil the steaks for about 4 minutes on one side, turn, and then grill for about 3 minutes on the other side. The time will vary with the thickness of the steaks.

Serve each tuna steak on a warmed plate with the relish and a lime wedge.

YIELD: 6 servings

SERVING SIZE: 1 tuna steak plus ¼ cup relish

Calories	Protein	Carbohydrates	Fat	Sodium
153	20 g	10 g	3.4 g	41 mg

Exchange: 3 lean meats; ½ fruit

Braised Salmon and Halibut Steaks

The advantage of using the two different fishes is that it provides varying tastes and is visually more pleasant, but the recipe works just as well with only salmon or halibut.

2 (8-ounce) salmon steaks
2 (8-ounce) halibut steaks
Unbleached flour for dusting the
    fish
2 tablespoons extra-virgin olive oil
½ cup Chicken Broth (page 133),
    Vegetable Broth (page 128), or
    low-fat, low-sodium canned broth
½ cup white wine
2 garlic cloves, minced
2 tablespoons chopped fresh oregano,
    or 1 teaspoon dried, crumbled

Salt substitute to taste
Ground white pepper to taste
3 shallots, finely minced
½ red bell pepper, cut into small dice
2 tablespoons unsalted, low-fat
    margarine
Radicchio leaves for garnish
Curly endive for garnish
Lime or lemon wedges for serving
2 tablespoons minced fresh parsley
    for garnish

Lightly dust the fish steaks with the flour. Heat the oil in a large nonstick skillet over medium heat. Sauté the steaks on both sides until golden brown.

Add the broth, white wine, garlic, oregano, salt substitute, white pepper, shallots, and bell pepper to the fish. Cover and cook over reduced heat. Periodically spoon the pan liquid over the fish. After about 5 minutes, toss the margarine in the pan and combine it with the liquid.

Cover and cook for about 3 minutes more. The fish should be done and resistant to the touch. Turn onto a warmed platter that you have garnished with the radicchio, endive, and lime wedges. Sprinkle the parsley over the fish and serve.

YIELD: 6 servings

SERVING SIZE: 2 ounces salmon; 2 ounces halibut

Calories	Protein	Carbohydrates	Fat	Sodium
222	25 g	2 g	10.67 g	153 mg

Exchange: 4 lean meats

Stir-fried Shrimp with Peas and Water Chestnuts

Your family will enjoy this delicious dish again and again, and you will enjoy it too because it is very quick and easy to make for those nights when you have about an hour to get dinner on the table. The things that you will need to do in advance are peel, devein, and marinate the shrimp, shell and blanch the peas if you use fresh ones, and have the rice cooked and ready to serve when the shrimp is done.

¾ pound medium shrimp (26 to 31 per pound), peeled and deveined

1½ cups shelled fresh or thawed frozen peas

2 teaspoons cornstarch

1 egg white

1 tablespoon dry sherry

½ teaspoon salt

Nonstick cooking spray for stir-frying

2 tablespoons finely minced garlic

1 bunch of green onions or scallions, cut into 2-inch lengths

3 tablespoons julienned fresh ginger

½ cup drained sliced low-sodium canned water chestnuts

1 small red bell pepper, stemmed, seeded, and julienned

3 cups cooked rice for serving

Rinse the shrimp under cold running water and pat them dry. Split each shrimp in half lengthwise, and then cut each of the halves in two, crosswise.

If using fresh peas, blanch them by dropping them in 3 cups of boiling water and boiling them for about 5 minutes, at which point they should be tender-crisp. Drain and run cold water over them to stop the cooking. This also helps them hold their color. If using thawed frozen peas, make sure they are fully thawed.

In a large bowl, toss the shrimp with the cornstarch until each shrimp is coated with the cornstarch. In a small bowl, whisk together the egg white, sherry, and salt and then stir this mixture into the shrimp and thoroughly combine. Cover and set the bowl in the refrigerator for 45 minutes to 1 hour.

Assemble all the ingredients so they are close at hand, as the cooking process takes only a matter of minutes. Remove the shrimp from the refrigerator.

Heat a wok, stir-fry pan, or large (10- or 12-inch) skillet over high heat. Lightly coat with the nonstick cooking spray and add the garlic, green onions, and ginger. Immediately drop the shrimp into the pan and stir-fry them for about 30 seconds. They should turn bright pink.

Drop in the peas, water chestnuts, and bell pepper and stir-fry them for about 1 minute to heat them through.

Remove the stir-fry from the pan and transfer to a platter. Serve at once with the hot rice.

YIELD: 6 servings   SERVING SIZE: ⅔ cup plus ½ cup rice

Calories	Protein	Carbohydrates	Fat	Sodium
158	15 g	23 g	2 g	182 mg

Exchange: 1 starch; 2 lean meats

Halibut Kebabs

Swordfish may be used for these kebabs, but it contains more sodium and fat than halibut. If you prefer not to use halibut, use any low-fat, low-sodium firm-fleshed fish, such as black drum, redfish, mahimahi, cod, whiting, or amberjack. This fish needs to rest in the marinade for at least 1 hour or up to 5 hours.

½ cup Chablis or other dry white wine

1 tablespoon plus 1 teaspoon canola
oil

5 tablespoons fresh lime or lemon
juice

¼ cup low-sodium Worcestershire
sauce

½ teaspoon coarsely ground black
pepper

3 large garlic cloves, minced

1 pound halibut, cut into 1-inch cubes

1 cup peeled, cored, and cubed fresh
pineapple or drained sugar-free
canned chunks

24 cherry tomatoes or firm, ripe
tomato chunks

1 large green bell pepper, stemmed,
seeded, and cut into 1-inch
cubes

1 large red bell pepper, stemmed,
seeded, and cut into 1-inch
cubes

24 snow peas, optional

24 pearl onions, ends trimmed and
peeled

24 small cremini or white
mushrooms

2 cups cooked rice for serving

In a large nonreactive bowl, whisk together the Chablis, 1 table-spoon of the oil, the lime juice, Worcestershire, black pepper, and garlic to blend. Add the fish and refrigerate from 1 to 5 hours.

Prepare the grill or heat the broiler. Drain the fish and save the marinade. Thread the fish on skewers alternating with the pineapple, tomatoes, green and red bell peppers, snow peas, if desired, onions, and mushrooms until 8 skewers are filled.

If using the grill, lightly oil it with the remaining teaspoon of oil. Arrange the kebabs on the grill or in the broiler. As you are cooking, be sure to brush the kebabs frequently with the marinade. Grill or broil until the fish is cooked through, being sure to turn the kebabs to cook on the other side at least once. The whole procedure should take 5 to 7 minutes.

Divide the rice equally among 4 plates and place 2 skewers on top of each bed of rice.

YIELD: 4 servings   SERVING SIZE: 2 kebabs plus ½ cup rice

Calories	Protein	Carbohydrates	Fat	Sodium
269	20 g	30 g	4.75 g	222 mg

Exchange: 2 lean meats; 1 starch; 1 fruit

Portuguese Fish Stew

When choosing the fish for the stew, you need to consider what is the freshest, the most reasonably priced, and, of course, the best-tasting. Suitable fishes for this dish are red or Pacific snapper, flounder, perch, black drum, or cod.

Serve this stew in a large, shallow bowl over either rice or noodles.

5 large red, Yukon Gold, or
  California white potatoes,
  unpeeled and quartered
6 cups fish broth, Chicken Broth
  (page 133), Garlic Broth (page
  132), Vegetable Broth (page
  128), or low-fat, low-sodium
  canned broth
¾ cup dry white wine
1½ cups diced yellow or white
  onions
4 large garlic cloves, minced
1 pound fresh fish, cut into medium
  pieces
Salt substitute to taste, optional

Ground white pepper to taste
4 to 5 ripe medium plum tomatoes,
  or 1 (14½-ounce) can low-sodium
  whole peeled plum tomatoes,
  coarsely chopped, with their juice
1 small red bell pepper, finely
  diced
6 to 7 kale leaves, stemmed and
  coarsely chopped
1 tablespoon fresh lime juice
1 to 1½ cups cooked basmati rice or
  noodles
2 tablespoons finely minced fresh
  parsley for garnish
Lime wedges for garnish

Place the potatoes in a large pot with boiling water and cook until they are tender but not falling apart, about 20 minutes.

While the potatoes are cooking, put the broth, wine, onions, and garlic into another large pot and over medium-high heat, bring to a boil. Cook the broth mixture for about 10 minutes and then add the fish. Simmer for about 7 minutes and add the salt substitute, if desired, and white pepper.

When the potatoes are done, thoroughly drain and add them to the fish mixture. Add the tomatoes and simmer for about 5 minutes.

Add the bell pepper, kale, and lime juice and cook for 8 to 10 minutes more.

Ladle into large bowls in which you have placed the hot rice. Garnish with the parsley and lime wedges. Serve.

YIELD: 6 servings   SERVING SIZE: ⅔ cup plus ¼ cup rice

Calories	Protein	Carbohydrates	Fat	Sodium
296	15 g	43 g	4.42 g	118 mg

Exchange: ½ lean meat; 2½ starches

Ceviche

This dish requires 3 to 4 hours of resting in the lime juice before serving. (See page 263 for more on marinating.) It can be made the night before you plan to serve it or most certainly the morning of serving, and it will hold in the refrigerator for 2 days. After the second day the vegetables tend to wilt and the fish will lose its firm texture.

Just as a marinade will tenderize as well as flavor foods, so will lime juice. In this traditional Mexican and southwestern way of fish preparation, the acid in the lime juice actually "cooks" the fish. You can watch the fish change from the translucent color of raw fish to the white, solid-looking color of "cooked" fish as it sits in the marinade.

1 pound flounder fillets, bay scallops, shrimp, or any firm-fleshed thin fillet
1 small red onion, finely diced
4 serrano chilies, or 2 jalapeño peppers, seeded and minced
Juice of 6 or 7 small limes, or as much as needed to cover the fish
1½ teaspoons salt

2 ripe plum tomatoes, diced
1 cup thinly sliced green onions or scallions
⅓ cup chopped fresh cilantro leaves
6 shredded romaine lettuce leaves for garnish
2 limes cut into fat wedges for garnish

Cut the fish into bite-size pieces and place in a large stainless steel or glass bowl. Add the red onion, chilies, and lime juice. Add the salt and mix thoroughly. Cover and refrigerate for at least 4 hours (3 hours if using scallops or shrimp).

After the fish turns white and is cooked, add the tomatoes, green onions, and cilantro. Stir to combine. To serve, drain as much liquid as possible from the ceviche, place on beds of shredded lettuce, and garnish with several lime wedges.

This dish also works beautifully as an appetizer (six 2-ounce [¼ cup] servings), served in crisp Bibb lettuce-leaf cups (see headnote, page 190).

YIELD: 4 servings as an entrée; 6 servings as an appetizer

SERVING SIZE: 3 ounces for entrée; 2 ounces for appetizer

Calories	Protein	Carbohydrates	Fat	Sodium
117	18.38 g	8.5 g	1.13 g	112.38 mg

Exchange: 3 lean meats; 1 vegetable

Tofu-and-Cheese-Stuffed Jumbo Shells

8 jumbo pasta shells

2 tablespoons finely grated peeled carrot

1½ tablespoons thinly sliced green onions or scallions

6 ounces tofu

⅓ cup low-fat ricotta cheese

⅓ cup shredded reduced-fat Monterey Jack cheese

⅓ cup shredded part-skim, reduced-fat mozzarella cheese

1 egg white, beaten

1 teaspoon toasted and crushed fennel seeds (see Note)

2 teaspoons sliced fresh basil, or ½ teaspoon dried, crumbled

½ teaspoon granulated garlic

½ teaspoon salt substitute

Coarsely ground black pepper to taste

3 cups warm Marinara Sauce (page 171) or Jiffy Marinara Sauce (page 173)

1 tablespoon finely minced fresh parsley for garnish, optional

Cook the pasta shells according to package directions and drain. Rinse with cold water and drain again. Set aside. Meanwhile, cook the carrot and green onions in a very small amount of water until tender. Drain.

In a medium bowl, mash the tofu with a fork and blend with the carrot mixture, ricotta, Monterey Jack, half of the mozzarella, and egg white. Add the fennel seeds, basil, granulated garlic, salt substitute, and pepper, making sure that the mixture is thoroughly combined.

Preheat the oven to 350°F.

Spread ⅓ cup of the sauce in an 8-inch square baking dish. Stuff each pasta shell with one-eighth of the tofu filling and place in the baking dish. Cover the shells with the remaining sauce and top with the rest of the mozzarella. Cover and heat in the oven for about 20 minutes, or until hot. Top with the parsley, if desired, and serve.

N O T E : To toast fennel seeds, place them in a dry skillet over medium heat and toss them until aromatic. Crush the seeds using a food processor or grinder, or crumble the seeds in your hands.

Y I E L D : 4 servings   S E R V I N G S I Z E : 2 shells

Calories	Protein	Carbohydrates	Fat	Sodium
285.25	14.95 g	28 g	8 g	181 mg

Exchange: 2 starches; 1½ medium-fat meats

Baked Chiles Rellenos

This recipe calls for poblano or Anaheim chili peppers. In making your choice, consider that the poblano chili is very spicy; the Anaheim is flavorful but not nearly as spicy. If these peppers are not available, you can substitute 10 bell peppers of any color. They are far less spicy, but they will work.

After the casserole has been put together, it needs to stand for at least 45 minutes. The casserole can be assembled the night before, covered, and refrigerated until baking the next day.

Nonstick cooking spray for the
   baking pan
12 large poblano or Anaheim chilies,
   roasted, peeled, split, and seeded
   (see page 264)
15 yellow corn tortillas, halved and
   sliced into ¼-inch-wide strips
2 cups thinly sliced yellow or white
   onions
¾ pound grated reduced-fat
   Monterey Jack cheese

The equivalent of 4 eggs in egg
   substitute, or 4 eggs
2 cups skim milk
1 tablespoon plus 1 teaspoon
   coarsely ground black pepper
2 tablespoons granulated garlic or
   garlic powder
2 teaspoons chili powder
½ teaspoon dried oregano, crumbled
½ teaspoon dried thyme, crumbled
½ teaspoon salt or salt substitute

Lightly coat an 8- or 9-inch square glass pan with the nonstick cooking spray. If you do not have a pan that size, use a 9-by-13-inch glass pan, which makes the casserole not quite so tall. If you do not have a glass pan, use a metal one, but increase the oven temperature to 375°F.

Arrange half of the chilies by opening and flattening them to completely cover the bottom of the baking dish. Arrange half of the tortillas evenly over the surface of the chilies and follow with a layer of half of the onions and then half of the cheese. Repeat the layering once more.

Beat together the eggs, milk, black pepper, granulated garlic, chili powder, oregano, salt, and thyme and pour the "custard" mixture over the casserole. Let stand refrigerated for at least 45 minutes.

Preheat the oven to 350°F.

Bake the chiles rellenos for about 1 hour or until golden brown and thoroughly set in the middle. Cool for 15 to 20 minutes. Slice and serve plain or with Ancho Chili Sauce (page 163), Pico de Gallo Salsa (page 170), or Tomatillo Sauce (page 165). The unused portion may be refrigerated for several days or may be frozen for future use.

YIELD: 6 servings SERVING SIZE: 1 (3-by-3-inch) piece

Calories	Protein	Carbohydrates	Fat	Sodium
356	22 g	42 g	12 g	196 mg

Exchange: 2½ starches; 1½ medium-fat meats; ½ milk; 1 fat

Desserts

Applesauce

Spicy Apple Slices

Pears Poached in Red Wine

Cardinal Peaches with Raspberries

Fruit Compote

Sweet Potato and Fresh Peach "Chantilly"

Strawberry-Almond Bread

Cranberry-Nut Bread

Basic Single Piecrust

Meringue Piecrust

Strawberry and Banana Yogurt Pie

"Slipped" Custard Pie

Sweet Potato Pie

Fresh Rhubarb and Strawberry Pie

Mixed Fruit Pie

Cardamom Cream Cake

Prune Puree

Steamed Chocolate Pudding

Chocolate Fudge Cake with Chocolate Icing

Spicy Applesauce Cake

Carrot Cake

Creole Rice Custard

Fresh Fruit Soufflé

Rice Pudding

Blueberry or Blackberry Pudding with
Lemon Wine Sauce

Sourdough Bread Pudding

Lime and Coconut Mousse

Orange, Grapefruit, and Raspberry Terrine

Chocolate Crepes

Cream Puffs

Vanilla Custard Cream

Applesauce

This applesauce is a very nice accompaniment to Rice Pudding (page 348), but it is also quite delicious on its own. If you wish to make a larger quantity, triple the amount of apples, add twice as much apple or orange juice, and double the amount of cinnamon. The amounts of nutmeg and lime juice are to taste and can easily be multiplied.

2 large tart apples, peeled, cored,
    and chopped into large chunks
¼ cup unsweetened natural apple or
    orange juice

¼ teaspoon ground cinnamon
Dash of ground nutmeg
½ teaspoon fresh lime or lemon
    juice

Combine all of the ingredients except the lime juice in a medium saucepan, bring to a boil, and simmer until the apples are soft. This should take about 10 to 12 minutes. Add the lime juice to the cooked apples, stir with a fork to break the apples down, and serve. May be kept, covered, in the refrigerator for a week or so.

YIELD: 2 cups

SERVING SIZE: ½ cup on its own;
2 tablespoons for rice pudding

Calories	Protein	Carbohydrates	Fat	Sodium
17	0 g	4 g	0 g	0 mg

Exchange: Free

Spicy Apple Slices

This is a quick and easy way to garnish and "spice up" your desserts. It turns a plain piece of cake or a bowl of Jell-O into something special. It even livens up something as delicious as Steamed Chocolate Pudding (page 337) and works beautifully as a filling for Chocolate Crepes (page 359).

The apples can be refrigerated before serving.

3 large apples (Granny Smith, Newton, Pippin, or Gala)
1 large lime or lemon
1 tablespoon granulated sugar substitute

1 teaspoon ground cinnamon
1 teaspoon vanilla extract
½ cup water
½ cup unsweetened natural apple juice

Core and thinly slice the apples. Grate the zest of the lime, then squeeze the lime juice into a small bowl. Pour the lime juice over the apples and toss to coat the apples. Set aside.

In a large (10- or 12-inch) skillet, whisk together the lime zest, sugar substitute, cinnamon, vanilla, water, and apple juice. Bring the mixture to a low boil over medium heat and whisk until the sugar substitute is completely dissolved.

Add the apple slices and poach until tender, about 3 minutes. Remove the apples from the syrup, cool, cover, and if you wish, refrigerate until ready to use. Discard the syrup or save it for some other use.

Use the apples for a filling or for a garnish.

YIELD: 2 cups   SERVING SIZE: ¼ cup

Calories	Protein	Carbohydrates	Fat	Sodium
37	0 g	10 g	0 g	0 mg

Exchange: ½ fruit

Pears Poached in Red Wine

This is a nice, easy dish for the fall and winter when pears are really at their best and least expensive. Pears prepared in this manner can be held in the refrigerator for 6 weeks to 2 months. I like to serve the poached pears chilled with a 3- to 4-ounce scoop of vanilla nonfat frozen yogurt in a large wineglass garnished with mint leaves.

It only takes about 20 to 25 minutes to poach the pears. They can be served warm or chilled. I like to poach the pears the night before or the morning of the day I want to serve them so that they have plenty of time to chill.

2 large limes or lemons

1 quart cold water

4 firm-fleshed, unblemished ripe
 medium pears

1½ cups red wine

2½ cups salt-free club soda or
 seltzer

1 orange, cut in half

1 tablespoon brown sugar substitute

1 (3-inch) cinnamon stick

½ teaspoon ground nutmeg

½ teaspoon ground allspice

6 to 7 whole cloves

1 quart vanilla nonfat yogurt,
 optional

Fresh mint leaves for garnish,
 optional

Squeeze the juice of 1 of the limes into the water. Carefully peel, halve, and core the pears to attain perfect halves. As you finish preparing each pear, put it in the bowl with the water and lime juice. This keeps the pears from discoloring.

In a large (3-quart) saucepan, combine the wine, club soda, the juice from 1 of the orange halves, and brown sugar substitute. Heat the poaching liquid and add the cinnamon stick, nutmeg, allspice, and cloves. Stir and bring the liquid to a simmer.

Cut the remaining lime and orange half into wedges. Drain the pears and add them to the poaching liquid. Add the lime and orange wedges, squeezing them as you put them into the liquid, and gently stir the whole mixture.

Cover and poach for 20 to 25 minutes. You may serve the pears at this point or chill them. If you are going to chill the pears, gently lift the pears from the saucepan and place them in a large bowl. Strain the liquid and cover the pears with it. Let the pears rest until they are cool, then cover and refrigerate.

When you are ready to serve, place each pear in a large wineglass. If you wish, put a 4-ounce scoop of frozen yogurt on top and garnish with the mint.

YIELD: 8 servings   SERVING SIZE: ½ pear

Calories	Protein	Carbohydrates	Fat	Sodium
74	15 g	12 g	0 g	20 mg

Exchange: 1 fruit

Cardinal Peaches with Raspberries

Cardamom is a delicious spice to use in poaching or in marinades. The dried fruit of a plant that belongs to the ginger family, it is very aromatic and has a slightly lemony aftertaste.

This is a quick and easy dish that requires a little poaching and some chilling (about 2 hours). It is a particularly good dish for the spring and summer when fresh, ripe peaches and raspberries abound.

3 large ripe, unblemished peaches
1½ quarts cold water
1 vanilla bean
1½ tablespoons plus 1 teaspoon
  granulated sugar substitute

¼ teaspoon ground cardamom
½ pint fresh raspberries
1 tablespoon blanched ground
  almonds, optional

Rinse the peaches and place them whole in a large (3- or 4-quart) saucepan.

In a medium bowl, combine the cold water, vanilla bean, 1½ table-spoons of the sugar substitute, and cardamom and pour into the saucepan, just covering the peaches.

Over medium-low heat, bring the mixture slowly to the simmering point and cover it. Simmer gently for 8 to 10 minutes.

Drain the peaches, and when they are cool enough to handle, slip off the skins.

Sprinkle the raspberries with the remaining teaspoon of sugar substitute and let them rest for about 15 minutes.

Puree the raspberries in a blender or small food processor. I never strain out the raspberry seeds, but if you wish to do so, you may press them through a small-meshed strainer at this point.

Cut the peaches in half and with a small paring knife, gently cut out the peach pit. Place the peach halves, cut side up, in a large bowl and cover each peach with some of the raspberry puree.

Cover the bowl with plastic wrap and chill the peaches until they are cold (several hours).

Place the peaches with the puree on 1 large serving dish or in individual bowls, sprinkle with the almonds, if desired, and serve.

YIELD: 6 peach halves   SERVING SIZE: 1 peach half
plus 2 to 3 tablespoons puree

Calories	Protein	Carbohydrates	Fat	Sodium
34	1 g	8 g	0 g	0 mg

Exchange: ½ fruit

Fruit Compote

The word *compote* comes from a French term for stewed fruit. It is usually served cold but can also be served warm (my preference) or at room temperature. After cooking, it has to cool to room temperature and be refrigerated before it can be served even if you plan to serve it warm. The flavors will fully develop during the refrigeration. This is a delightful way to serve the fresh fruit of the season. It works well as a light dessert, but leftovers can also be served as an accompaniment to fish, meat, or poultry. It will keep in the refrigerator for at least 1 week.

1¼ pounds fresh peaches, plums, apples, or pears, washed, peeled, cored or pitted, and cut into fairly large (about 1-inch) dice (about 2 cups)

1 cup cold water

¼ teaspoon salt

¼ cup granulated brown sugar substitute or Sucanat

1 teaspoon grated lime or lemon zest

2 teaspoons fresh lime or lemon juice

⅛ teaspoon ground white pepper

¼ teaspoon ground cinnamon

⅛ teaspoon ground allspice

Dash of ground cloves

Dash of ground cardamom

2 tablespoons brandy

In a large (3-quart), heavy saucepan, combine all of the ingredients and bring to a boil over high heat.

As soon as the mixture begins to boil, cover and reduce the heat just enough to keep a very low simmer going.

Simmer for about 25 minutes, until the fruit is tender but not mushy.

Remove the pan from the heat, pour the mixture into a stainless steel or glass bowl, and allow it to cool to room temperature. After it cools, cover it with a lid or plastic wrap and refrigerate.

To serve the compote at room temperature, remove it from the refrigerator 25 to 30 minutes before serving. If you prefer it warm, reheat it in a small skillet just before serving.

YIELD: 5 servings   SERVING SIZE: ½ cup

Calories	Protein	Carbohydrates	Fat	Sodium
41	0 g	8 g	0 g	51 mg

Exchange: ½ fruit

Sweet Potato and Fresh Peach "Chantilly"

I put *chantilly* in quotation marks here because traditionally the word is used when one adds whipped cream to a dish. In this dessert, I am adding a nondairy whipped cream substitute right before serving. This is a very tasty and unusual combination. It has the added advantage of being rather inexpensive.

The sweet potatoes need to be baked in a very hot oven (about 450°F) for 30 to 35 minutes. After they have cooled, they can be peeled and diced. The peaches need to be peeled, pitted, and diced.

Nonstick cooking spray for the
   baking pan
4 medium sweet potatoes, roasted
   (see headnote), peeled, and diced
   into ¾-inch cubes (about 2 cups)
1¼ pounds firm, ripe peaches,
   peeled, pitted, and diced into ¾-
   inch cubes (about 2 cups)

⅓ cup cold water
2 teaspoons liquid sugar
   substitute
2 teaspoons fresh lime or lemon
   juice
Dash of salt substitute
¼ teaspoon ground white pepper
2 tablespoons brandy

4 tablespoons unsalted, low-fat
  margarine
½ teaspoon ground cinnamon
¼ teaspoon ground nutmeg

¼ teaspoon ground cardamom
1 cup nonfat, nondairy whipped
  topping

Preheat the oven to 375°F. Lightly coat a 1½- or 2-quart baking dish with the nonstick cooking spray.

In a large (3- or 4-quart), heavy-bottomed saucepan, combine the sweet potatoes and peaches with the water, liquid sugar substitute, lime juice, salt substitute, white pepper, and brandy. Bring to a boil over medium heat and simmer for 8 to 10 minutes. You will want the liquid in the pan to be thickened.

Remove the sweet potatoes and peaches from the saucepan and put half of them into the prepared baking dish. Pour some of the syrup from the saucepan over the layer in the baking dish. Cut a little less than half of the margarine into small pieces and dot the layer with it. Sprinkle with half of the cinnamon, nutmeg, and cardamom.

Add the remainder of the sweet potatoes and peaches and cover with the rest of the syrup from the saucepan. Sprinkle with the remaining cinnamon, nutmeg, and cardamom. Dot with the rest of the margarine.

Bake, uncovered, for about 35 minutes. At this point the liquid in the baking dish should be very thick and the top should be brown. Top each serving with 2 tablespoons of the nondairy whipped topping.

YIELD: 8 servings   SERVING SIZE: ½ cup

Calories	Protein	Carbohydrates	Fat	Sodium
130	1.2 g	23 g	3 g	35 mg

Exchange: 1½ fruits; ½ fat

Strawberry-Almond Bread

This recipe makes 1 miniloaf of bread, 8 inches by 4 inches, rather than the standard 9-by-5-inch loaf. The recipe can easily be doubled to make 2 miniloaves if you are entertaining or if you want to give 1 loaf away. I prefer to make this recipe in the smaller loaf pan because the smaller size makes it easier to arrange the slices on a cake plate and it is such a rich bread that it is wiser to eat it in moderation.

Nonstick cooking spray for the loaf pan

4 tablespoons unsalted, low-fat margarine

¼ cup granulated sugar substitute

1½ teaspoons vanilla extract

The equivalent of 2 eggs in egg substitute, or 2 eggs

1½ cups all-purpose flour

½ teaspoon salt substitute

A rounded ¼ teaspoon cream of tartar

¼ teaspoon baking soda

½ cup sugar-free, low-sodium strawberry jam

¼ cup sour cream substitute

Grated zest and juice of ½ lime or lemon

¼ cup blanched sliced almonds

Preheat the oven to 340°F. Coat an 8-by-4-inch loaf pan with the nonstick cooking spray.

In a large bowl with an electric mixer, cream the margarine and the sugar substitute until light and somewhat fluffy. Add the vanilla.

If you are using egg substitute, beat it in a separate bowl and then gradually add it to the creamed mixture as you beat well. If you are using whole eggs, add them one at a time, beating well after each addition.

Sift together the flour, salt substitute, cream of tartar, and baking soda. Whisk together the jam, sour cream substitute, and lime zest and juice.

Add the jam mixture alternately with the flour mixture to the creamed mixture, stirring to combine. Stir in the almonds.

Pour the batter into the prepared loaf pan and bake for 40 to 45 minutes, until the bread is firm in the center.

Cool on a rack for about 10 minutes before removing from the pan. Cut and serve.

YIELD: 1 (8-by-4-inch) loaf   SERVING SIZE: 1 (1-inch) slice

Calories	Protein	Carbohydrates	Fat	Sodium
68	2 g	9 g	5 g	50 mg

Exchange: ½ starch; 1 fat

Cranberry-Nut Bread

This is a delicious fruit bread that is great anytime, not only during the holidays. If you are using frozen berries they don't need to be thawed; just rinse them, drain them well, and pop them in the batter.

After baking the bread and cooling it, chill the bread for about 2 hours before serving.

Nonstick cooking spray for the loaf pan

2 cups all-purpose flour plus 1 tablespoon for dusting the pan

1½ cups very coarsely chopped fresh or frozen cranberries (see headnote)

¼ cup blanched sliced almonds

1 tablespoon grated orange zest

2 teaspoons grated lime zest

¼ cup granulated sugar substitute

1½ teaspoons baking powder

½ teaspoon salt substitute

½ teaspoon baking soda

2 tablespoons solid vegetable shortening

¾ cup fresh orange juice or juice made from frozen unsweetened concentrate

The equivalent of 1 egg in egg substitute, thoroughly beaten

Preheat the oven to 350°F.

Thoroughly spray a 9-by-5-inch loaf pan with the nonstick cooking spray. Dust the pan with 1 tablespoon of the flour.

In a large bowl, combine the cranberries, almonds, and orange and lime zest and set aside.

In another large bowl, mix together the 2 cups of flour, the sugar substitute, baking powder, salt substitute, and baking soda. Cut in the shortening using 2 forks. Stir in the orange juice and the egg substitute, mixing to moisten the dry mixture.

Fold in the cranberry mixture, being sure to thoroughly combine.

Spoon the batter into the prepared pan and bake for about 60 minutes. The bread is done when it is firm in the middle and when a toothpick or cake tester inserted in the middle comes out clean.

Cool on a rack for about 20 minutes. Remove from the pan and cool completely. Wrap, refrigerate until chilled, and serve.

YIELD: 1 (9-by-5-inch) loaf   SERVING SIZE: 1 (1-inch) slice

Calories	Protein	Carbohydrates	Fat	Sodium
88	2 g	14 g	5 g	76 mg

Exchange: ½ starch; ½ fruit; 1 fat

Basic Single Piecrust

I know, I know, you are thinking that you can't make good piecrusts. In fact, I can hear you now: "But I can't make piecrust!" Nonsense. Anyone can make good piecrust. This is one of those instances when just a little bit more is too much. *Do not* handle the dough too much when combining it. If you overmix the flour and the shortening together, you eliminate the pockets of shortening that should form between the layers of flour, water, and lemon juice and you will not achieve a flaky crust. *Do not* use too much flour when rolling out the dough. *Do not* roll the dough too much.

You need to use cold or chilled ingredients when making the dough.

To keep the shortening chilled when measuring it is easiest to measure using cold water. Fill a 1-cup glass measuring cup with ⅓ cup cold water, add shortening until the water rises to the ⅔-cup measuring line, and you have ⅓ cup of shortening. Not only does the shortening stay cold, the measuring cup is very easy to clean.

1 cup plus 1 tablespoon all-purpose flour	*⅓ cup chilled shortening*
	1½ tablespoons ice water
Dash of salt	*2¼ teaspoons chilled lemon juice*

To mix the dough by hand: in a large bowl, cut the shortening into small chunks and toss it lightly in the flour to coat. Keep tossing and blending the mixture with your fingers, picking up more flour as you mix, until the dough feels like very coarse bread crumbs. Then, sprinkle the water and lemon juice over the flour mixture and work the liquids into the dough until the dough is just barely moistened. (If, in spite of all of your efforts, you feel that the pastry dough may be overblended, you can add a few splashes of apple cider vinegar to the dough before you chill it, which will help tenderize the flour during the baking process.) Form the dough into a ball, wrap it in plastic wrap, and chill it for about half an hour before rolling it out. It is important to chill the dough even if you do not live in a warm climate.

Place the chilled ball of dough in the center of a lightly dusted rolling surface (use no more than 2 tablespoons of flour at most), flatten it a bit with the heel of your hand, and roll the crust from the center in short, quick strokes. Roll the dough for the bottom crust about 1½ inches larger than the pie pan and about ⅛ inch thick. For a top crust, roll the dough about 2 inches larger than the pie pan and a little thinner. You can either loosely roll up the crust onto the rolling pin to move it to line the pie pan or place the pie pan upside down on top of the crust and with a spatula, very gently lift the dough from the underside and turn the pan right side up.

To help ensure a flaky, golden brown crust while the pie is baking, I always use glass pie pans so I can see what the crust looks like, and I always bake on the bottom shelf of the oven. I never put a pie pan directly on top of a cookie sheet. If I'm worried that the filling will leak out, I put a cookie sheet on the bottom of the oven itself. The oven stays cleaner and the crust will not be soggy.

Remember, when you use glass baking dishes in the oven, lower the baking or roasting temperature by 25 degrees, as glass tends to distribute heat more rapidly than metal does. This also minimizes the possibility of having a soggy crust.

So, don't overmix, overwork, or overbake, bake in glass on the bottom shelf of the oven, and you will have good piecrusts.

FOOD PROCESSOR PREPARATION

Because my mother makes the best piecrust I have ever eaten and makes her pie dough in a food processor, this is my favorite method also. It is much faster than by hand and she swears it is foolproof.

To mix the dough using the food processor: put all the ingredients in the bowl of the food processor with the steel blade in place. Using the pulse button, blend the dough for about 10 to 15 seconds, adding a bit more ice water if the dough is too dry. Quickly shape the dough into a ball, wrap it in plastic wrap, and chill it. Roll out the dough and bake as directed above.

YIELD: 1 (9-inch) piecrust, to be divided into 8 wedges

Meringue Piecrust

This is a quick and easy crust recipe that works beautifully with lime or lemon pies and cream pies. You might also want to fill this crust with softened nonfat frozen yogurt topped with fresh fruit or simply with fresh fruit. It has the advantage of having no fat, and as it is made with egg whites, it is low in cholesterol and calories. The only fat is that used to oil the pan in which the meringue is baked.

Meringues are handled differently from other baked goods. Baking meringues is really more of a drying process than a heating process, as a very low heat is used. The heat should always be a bottom heat, not a top heat. After you have baked the crust for the desired amount of time, do not remove the pie pan from the oven until the oven is cold.

4 egg whites, at room temperature (about 75°F)
1 teaspoon vanilla extract
⅛ teaspoon cream of tartar

1 cup granulated sugar substitute, sifted through a fine-mesh strainer
Nonstick cooking spray for the pie pan

The temperature of the oven determines the texture of the meringue. For a soft, crunchy meringue, preheat the oven to 225°F. For a chewier meringue, preheat the oven to 275°F. If you want a texture literally somewhere in-between (not quite so soft and a little chewy), preheat the oven to 250°F. I generally preheat the oven to 250°F, as it seems to give me the texture that is the most versatile.

In a large bowl with an electric mixer, beat the egg whites until they are foamy and then add the vanilla and cream of tartar.

Continue to beat the mixture and add the sugar substitute, several tablespoons at a time. The egg white mixture must be constantly beaten until all of the sugar is added. The mixture should be thick and glossy and stand in very stiff, but not dry, peaks. Be careful not to overbeat.

Thoroughly coat a 9-inch metal or glass pie pan with the nonstick cooking spray (if glass is used, lower the oven temperature 25 degrees). Turn the meringue into the pie pan, spread it evenly over the bottom of the pan, and gently bring it up the sides in fairly evenly spaced peaks.

Bake for about 1 hour. The meringue should be solid but should have no color. Turn off the oven and let the oven cool completely before removing the pie pan.

Fill the shell and serve. If you are going to save the shell, save at room temperature in an airtight container.

YIELD: 1 (9-inch) piecrust

For entire piecrust:				
Calories	Protein	Carbohydrates	Fat	Sodium
60	12 g	0 g	0 g	200 mg

Exchange: Free

Strawberry and Banana Yogurt Pie

This is a perfect filling for the Meringue Piecrust. It's quick and easy and the resulting pie is one your family will want again and again. In the winter substitute IQF (individually quick-frozen) raspberries for the strawberries. In fact, any combination of fruits may be used to combine with the yogurt. Experiment a bit and see what tastes good to you.

I usually buy yogurt in the quart size as I use it a lot and it is less expensive this way.

2 pints fresh ripe strawberries

24 ounces plain nonfat yogurt (3 cups)

1 large ripe banana, cut into chunks

1 tablespoon granulated sugar substitute

1 teaspoon fresh lime or lemon juice

1 cup nonfat, nondairy whipped topping (follow package directions for mixing), chilled

1 baked 9-inch Meringue Piecrust (page 322), cooled

Fresh mint leaves for garnish, optional

Rinse, drain, and hull the strawberries. Set aside one-third of the strawberries for garnishing the pie when it is finished. Slice the remaining two-thirds of the strawberries.

Put one-third (8 ounces) of the yogurt into a blender. Add the banana and the sugar substitute. Blend until all of the ingredients are incorporated. Set aside in a large bowl.

Put the remaining two-thirds of the yogurt into the blender and add one-third of the sliced strawberries and the lime juice. Blend until completely incorporated. Add the strawberry yogurt mixture to the banana yogurt in the bowl along with the whipped topping. Whisk until thoroughly combined.

Stir the remaining one-third of the sliced strawberries into the mixture in the bowl and pour the entire mixture into the pie shell.

Slice the remaining reserved whole strawberries in half lengthwise, place them on the pie, and serve. Garnish with the fresh mint leaves, if desired.

YIELD: 1 (9-inch) pie   SERVING SIZE: ⅛ pie

Calories	Protein	Carbohydrates	Fat	Sodium
106	8 g	17 g	0 g	90 mg

Exchange: 1 milk; ½ fruit

"Slipped" Custard Pie

This is a great pie — it's not difficult to make and because of the method used in preparation, you are assured a nice crisp crust. This old-fashioned method keeps the piecrust flaky and the custard extremely smooth and silky. You will need 2 pie pans exactly the same size and shape. I like to use a glass pie pan to bake the custard, which I then "slip" into the prebaked pie shell. If you are not going to serve the pie right away, refrigerate the custard separately and don't combine the custard and crust until you are ready to serve. The custard may be made a day or so in advance.

Garnish the pie slices with fresh fruit; use sliced strawberries or raspberries in the spring and summertime, and peeled, sliced kiwis in the fall and winter.

1 (9-inch) Basic Single Piecrust (page 319)
Nonstick cooking spray for the pie pan used for baking the custard
6 tablespoons granulated sugar substitute
¼ teaspoon salt
½ teaspoon ground cardamom
2½ cups 1% milk, lightly scalded
2 teaspoons vanilla extract
The equivalent of 4 eggs in egg substitute, beaten
Fresh fruit for garnish (see headnote)

Preheat the oven to 415°F if using a 9-inch metal pie pan and 390°F if using a 9-inch glass one.

Roll the prepared piecrust to about ⅛ inch thick. Line the pie pan with the piecrust, leaving about a 1-inch overhang of dough. Fold the overhang under and flute to make a decorative edge. Prick the dough all over with the tines of a fork, place the pan in the middle of the bottom shelf of the oven, and bake the dough for 15 to 17 minutes, until the shell is lightly browned. Remove from the oven and set aside.

Lower the oven thermostat to 350°F for a metal pie pan and 325°F for a glass one. With the nonstick cooking spray, coat a pie pan the same size and shape as the baked pie shell.

In a large bowl, combine the sugar substitute, salt, cardamom, milk, and vanilla. Whisk in the egg substitute and mix well. Pour the mixture through a fine-meshed strainer and whisk again. Pour the mixture into the prepared pan and then set the pan in a larger pan filled with about ½ inch of hot water.

Bake the custard for about 35 to 40 minutes. The custard should barely be set. You need to be careful not to overbake the custard or it will be watery.

Remove the pan of custard from its water bath in the oven and set it on a rack to cool. If you are not going to serve the pie right away, refrigerate the custard. You need to put the pie together as close to serving time as possible for the crust to stay crisp.

Run a sharp knife around the edge of the custard and shake the pan gently to loosen the custard from the bottom of the pan. Hold the pan with the custard over the pie shell and ease the filling very gingerly into the shell. Once you've "slipped" the custard into the pie shell, gently shake the shell to help it settle into place. Cut into 8 servings, garnish with the fruit, and serve.

YIELD: 1 (9-inch) pie   SERVING SIZE: ⅛ pie

Calories	Protein	Carbohydrates	Fat	Sodium
190	6 g	14 g	12 g	105 mg

Exchange: ½ starch; ½ milk; 2 fats

Sweet Potato Pie

Sweet potatoes and yams are not of the same botanical genus but usually can be used interchangeably. However, some species of yams contain harmful chemicals, so yams should never be eaten raw, whereas sweet potatoes can be.

In a pinch, canned unsalted, unsweetened sweet potatoes can be used instead of freshly roasted potatoes. They must be thoroughly drained and rolled in layers of paper towels to remove any excess moisture.

Roast washed sweet potatoes or yams in a preheated 450°F oven for about 1 hour. Cool the potatoes, then peel them and cut out any dark spots. Cut the potatoes into large chunks and mash them either with a big spoon or with a potato masher. To bake the potatoes in the microwave, prick them with a fork, place them on paper towels, and cook for about 21 minutes, or according to the manufacturer's instructions.

1 (9-inch) Basic Single Piecrust (page 319)	½ teaspoon ground cinnamon
3 cooked medium sweet potatoes or yams, mashed (1½ cups)	¼ teaspoon ground nutmeg
	The equivalent of 2 eggs in egg substitute, beaten
½ cup brown sugar substitute	1 cup skim or 1% milk
½ teaspoon salt	1½ teaspoons vanilla extract
A heaping ¼ teaspoon ground allspice	½ teaspoon fresh lime or lemon juice

Roll the prepared piecrust to about ⅛ inch thick. Line a 9-inch glass pie pan with the piecrust, leaving a 1-inch overhang of dough. Fold the overhang under and flute to make a decorative edge.

Preheat the oven to 425°F.

In a large bowl, combine the sweet potatoes with the brown sugar substitute, salt, allspice, cinnamon, nutmeg, egg substitute, milk, vanilla, and lime juice.

Mix thoroughly and pour into the pie shell and bake for 15 minutes.

Reduce the oven temperature to 325°F and bake for 30 to 35 minutes more. A knife inserted in the center of the pie filling should come out clean.

Serve immediately or chill and serve.

YIELD: 1 (9-inch) pie   SERVING SIZE: ⅛ pie

Calories	Protein	Carbohydrates	Fat	Sodium
173	4 g	25 g	8.28 g	145 mg

Exchange: 1½ starches; 1 fat

Fresh Rhubarb and Strawberry Pie

The combination of fresh rhubarb and fresh strawberries cannot be beaten. The sharp, distinctive flavor of rhubarb is a perfect counterpoint to the sweet, succulent flavor of ripe strawberries. Rhubarb is very low in fat (less than one-tenth of a gram per ½ cup) and calories and has good dietary fiber.

This pie is delicious when topped with seasoned nonfat yogurt or with nonfat, nondairy whipped topping.

The piecrust for this pie needs to be baked in advance, and the pie needs to stand for several hours at room temperature or in the refrigerator before serving.

1 (9-inch) *Basic Single Piecrust* (page 319)

2 cups sliced rhubarb (about 4 large stalks)

⅓ cup plus 1 teaspoon granulated sugar substitute

1 cup unsweetened natural apple juice

3½ tablespoons cornstarch dissolved in ⅓ cup cold water

2 cups rinsed, hulled, and sliced ripe strawberries

1 cup plain nonfat yogurt

1 teaspoon finely grated lime zest

1 teaspoon fresh lime or lemon juice

Preheat the oven to 415° F if using a metal pie pan and 390° F if using a glass pie pan.

Roll the prepared piecrust to ⅛ inch thick. Line a 9-inch pie pan with the piecrust, leaving a 1-inch overhang of dough. Fold the overhang under and flute to make a decorative edge. Prick the crust all over with the tines of a fork and bake for about 25 minutes. The crust should be golden. Allow the crust to cool to room temperature before filling it.

Put the rhubarb, ⅓ cup of the sugar substitute, and the apple juice in a large (3-quart) saucepan and bring the mixture to a boil over medium heat, stirring until the sugar substitute is completely dissolved. Reduce the heat and continue to cook at a simmer for about 6 to 7 minutes more, at which point the rhubarb should be tender-crisp.

Stir the dissolved cornstarch thoroughly and place in a medium bowl. Set the mixture aside.

Add the strawberries to the rhubarb mixture in the saucepan and cook until both the rhubarb and the strawberries are tender, about 2 to 3 minutes. Add ¼ cup of the hot liquid from this mixture to the dissolved cornstarch and quickly stir it with a fork.

Add this cornstarch mixture to the saucepan, blend thoroughly, and over a low simmering heat, continue cooking, stirring constantly, until the mixture thickens and loses some of its cloudiness. This should take about 5 to 6 minutes.

Remove the pan from the heat and pour the mixture into the cooled, prebaked crust. Allow to stand for several hours at room temperature or in the refrigerator before serving.

Just before serving, whisk together the yogurt, the remaining teaspoon of sugar substitute, lime zest, and lime juice. To serve, cut the pie into 8 slices and top each piece with about 2 tablespoons of the yogurt mixture.

YIELD: 1 (9-inch) pie   SERVING SIZE: ⅛ pie

Calories	Protein	Carbohydrates	Fat	Sodium
168	3 g	19 g	8.5 g	22 mg

Exchange: 1 starch; ¼ fruit; 1½ fats

Mixed Fruit Pie

For this pie, there are many fabulous fruit combinations that work just beautifully. I like the taste sensation of apple and blackberry, apple and peach, peach and blackberry, blackberry and blueberry, or blueberry and apple.

Blackberries are an interesting fruit, and in this country many different berries are known by the name blackberry. The skin color ranges from green to red to black as the fruit ripens, and all three stages are found on any one plant in late August and early September. In the Midwest, loganberries are called blackberries, and in Texas, Brazosberries are often called blackberries. But the real thing is either conical or oval in shape and can be up to 1 inch long. They do beautifully in pies and cobblers but do need a squeeze of fresh lime or lemon juice to sharpen their taste. Berries also require less sugar than other fruits, so if you make the pie with berries only, add less sugar substitute than the recipe calls for.

2 (9-inch) Basic Single Piecrust recipes (page 319)

6 cups rinsed, peeled, and sliced fresh fruit (berries do not need to be sliced)

¼ cup granulated sugar substitute (approximately)

3½ to 4 tablespoons all-purpose flour

1 teaspoon finely grated lime or lemon zest

1 tablespoon fresh lime or lemon juice

½ teaspoon ground cinnamon or ground nutmeg

1 tablespoon low-fat margarine, optional

¼ cup skim milk

Preheat the oven to 390°F if using a metal pie pan and 365°F if using a glass pie pan.

Roll 1 of the prepared piecrusts to ⅛ inch thick. Line a 9-inch pie pan with the piecrust, leaving a ½-inch overhang of dough. Roll out the remaining piecrust a bit thinner than ⅛ inch and set it aside.

In a large bowl, combine the fruit with the sugar substitute, flour, lime zest, lime juice, and cinnamon. Toss until the fruit is coated with the sugar substitute and flour, and the zest and cinnamon are evenly distributed. Let the mixture rest for at least 12 minutes but not more than 15 minutes.

Turn the fruit mixture into the crust, dot with the margarine, if desired, and pour the skim milk over all of it.

Gently place the top crust over the filling and fold the top crust over the bottom. Crimp together the edges to seal, and flute to make a decorative edge. Cut about six 2-inch slits in the top crust so that the steam can escape.

Bake on the bottom shelf of the oven for about 50 minutes, until the crust is golden brown and the filling is bubbling.

YIELD: 1 (9-inch) pie   SERVING SIZE: ⅛ pie

Calories	Protein	Carbohydrates	Fat	Sodium
301	3 g	33 g	18 g	9 mg

Exchange: 1 starch; 1 fruit; 3 fats

NOTE: If you wish to reduce the amount of fat grams in this dessert, you can make this pie with a single crust and add a nonfat whipped topping. This reduces the fat grams to 10, the fat exchange to about 1.3, and the calories to 181.

Cardamom Cream Cake

This cake is light, fragrant, and delicious. Cardamom is one of my favorite spices and works beautifully in this dessert. Its lemony taste is further enhanced by the addition of the lemon juice and zest.

Nonstick cooking spray for the tube
   pan
2 cups all-purpose flour plus 1½ to
   2 tablespoons for dusting the pan
6 tablespoons granulated sugar
   substitute
2 teaspoons baking powder
1½ teaspoons ground cardamom
½ teaspoon salt
The equivalent of 3 eggs in egg
   substitute, at room temperature

2 lemons
½ cup sour cream substitute or
   plain nonfat yogurt
½ cup 2% milk
Unsweetened natural apple juice to
   equal ½ cup when added to the
   juice of one lemon
¼ cup confectioners' sugar
   substitute for "icing" garnish

Preheat the oven to 350°F. Coat a 9-inch tube pan with the nonstick cooking spray and lightly dust with 1½ to 2 tablespoons of the flour.

In a large bowl with an electric mixer, combine the 2 cups of flour, the sugar substitute, baking powder, cardamom, and salt on a low speed. Blend in the egg substitute at a low speed and mix thoroughly.

Meanwhile, finely grate the zest from 1 of the lemons to equal 1 tablespoon. Squeeze the lemon and combine the juice with enough apple juice to make ½ cup of liquid. In a small bowl, mix the sour cream substitute, milk, lemon and apple juices, and the tablespoon of lemon zest, making sure that everything is thoroughly combined.

Add the sour cream mixture to the flour mixture at high speed and continue to beat at that speed. As you are mixing the cake, scrape the sides of the bowl with a rubber spatula and continue to beat until the texture is like softly whipped cream.

Turn the batter into the prepared pan. Bake in the middle of the oven for 55 to 60 minutes. At this point the cake should test done. (Insert a wooden skewer or a cake tester in the highest part of the cake; if the skewer comes out clean, the cake is done.)

Cool the cake in the pan for about 5 minutes, then invert on a cooling rack and cool completely before removing from the pan.

Remove the cake from the pan, put it on a plate, and slice it into serving pieces. Slice the remaining lemon into thin rounds. Sift a few teaspoons of the confectioners' sugar substitute over each piece and add a lemon round. To make the lemon round look a bit fancier, you can slice it from the outside rim to the center and twist it.

YIELD: 1 (9-inch) tube cake   SERVING SIZE: 1 (2-inch) slice

Calories	Protein	Carbohydrates	Fat	Sodium
113	4 g	19 g	2 g	134 mg

Exchange: 1 starch; ¼ fruit

Prune Puree

It is becoming quite popular in cooking circles to use prunes to "prune" the fats from many recipes. The rule of thumb is to use prune puree in a direct one-to-one substitution for any fat (butter, margarine, or oil) you would use in baked goods; for example, ½ cup of margarine would be replaced with ½ cup of prune puree.

This use of prunes cuts the fat by at least 75 percent and the calories by about 25 percent, and takes the cholesterol count to zero. Prunes also add a measurable nutritional boost in that they contain dietary fiber, iron, vitamin A, and potassium.

Prune puree works best in recipes you don't expect to come out crisp, such as brownies and brownielike cakes. Adding prune puree deepens the intensity of their flavor and texture. It works especially well with baked chocolate goods, and also with Carrot Cake (page 343).

You can buy prune butter and use it in the same way you would prune puree, but it is so simple and inexpensive to make the puree that there is no reason to buy the prepared product.

All you need are pitted prunes, water or apple juice, vanilla, and a food processor.

> *1 cup natural, unsweetened pitted prunes*
> *2 teaspoons vanilla extract*
> *6 tablespoons water or unsweetened natural*
> *   apple juice*

In the bowl of a food processor, combine the prunes and vanilla. Begin processing, adding the water slowly through the feed tube. Continue with the processing until the mixture is smooth. Use as needed, storing the unused amount in the refrigerator, tightly covered.

YIELD: 1¼ cups

For ¼ cup of puree:

Calories	Protein	Carbohydrates	Fat	Sodium
45	0.4 g	12 g	0 g	0.8 mg

Exchange: Free

Steamed Chocolate Pudding

This chocolate pudding is sweet, moist, and delicious. It also has a secret ingredient — prunes. Prune puree and unsweetened cocoa give you the tastes you crave and eliminate many of the fats you certainly do not need.

This recipe may be easily halved or doubled.

Nonstick cooking spray for the
   pudding mold
½ cup unsweetened cocoa
¼ cup Prune Puree made with apple
   juice (page 336)
½ cup evaporated skim milk
¼ cup granulated sugar substitute
The equivalent of 1 egg in egg
   substitute

1 teaspoon vanilla extract
1 cup all-purpose flour
1 teaspoon lemon zest
½ teaspoon ground cardamom
1½ teaspoons baking powder
¼ teaspoon salt

Coat a 1-quart pudding mold with the nonstick cooking spray.

Set a rack inside a fairly tall stockpot or Dutch oven. If you don't have a rack that will fit inside a pot, put an ovenproof pie pan upside down in the pot and cover it with water (about 4 to 5 inches of water). Cover the pot and bring the water to a boil, lowering the heat to keep the water at a very low simmer.

In a large mixing bowl, whisk together the cocoa, prune puree, half of the evaporated skim milk, the sugar substitute, and egg substitute. Whisk together thoroughly and add the vanilla.

In a small bowl, combine the flour, lemon zest, cardamom, baking powder, and salt. Add along with the remaining half of the evaporated skim milk to the cocoa mixture. Whisk together so that the mixture is thoroughly combined.

Pour the mixture into the prepared mold. Set on the rack or on the inverted pie pan inside the pot of boiling water. Be sure that the water comes at least halfway up the side of the mold. If there is not enough water, more boiling water should be added.

Cover the pot and steam the pudding for about 45 minutes.

Serve the pudding either hot or cold with fresh fruit, Fruit Compote (page 312), or Spicy Apple Slices (page 308). Unused pudding may be wrapped tightly and stored in the refrigerator.

YIELD: 12 servings   SERVING SIZE: 1 slice

Calories	Protein	Carbohydrates	Fat	Sodium
63	3 g	10 g	1 g	73 mg

Exchange: ½ milk; ½ fruit

Chocolate Fudge Cake with Chocolate Icing

This cake owes its lack of fat to prune puree. The intensity of the chocolate flavor will both surprise and delight you.

Cake

Nonstick cooking spray for the
  baking pan
½ cup water
½ cup unsweetened natural apple
  juice
½ cup Prune Puree made with apple
  juice (page 336)
3 large egg whites
2 teaspoons vanilla extract

1 cup plus 2 tablespoons all-purpose
  flour
3 tablespoons granulated sugar
  substitute
¾ cup unsweetened cocoa powder
1½ teaspoons baking powder
¼ teaspoon baking soda
¼ teaspoon salt

Icing

2½ cups confectioners' sugar
  substitute
¼ cup unsweetened cocoa
  powder

¼ cup 1% milk
½ teaspoon vanilla
  extract

To make the cake, preheat the oven to 350°F. Coat a 9-inch square baking pan with the nonstick cooking spray.

In a large bowl with an electric mixer, thoroughly combine the water, apple juice, prune puree, egg whites, and vanilla. Be sure that the mixture is well blended.

Add the flour, sugar substitute, cocoa powder, baking powder, baking soda, and salt and completely mix.

Pour the batter into the prepared baking pan. Tap the pan on a hard surface several times to remove any air bubbles and bake for about 30 minutes, until a skewer inserted in the middle of the cake comes out clean. Set on a rack to cool completely and then remove the cake from the pan.

Meanwhile, prepare the icing: combine the confectioners' sugar substitute, cocoa powder, milk, and vanilla in a 1-quart bowl and with an electric mixer, beat until the icing is completely smooth.

Spread the icing on the cake after the cake has been removed from the pan. Cut into 3-inch squares and serve.

YIELD: 1 cake (9 servings)   SERVING SIZE: 1 (3-by-3-inch) square

For the cake without the icing:

Calories	Protein	Carbohydrates	Fat	Sodium
91	4 g	16 g	0 g	123 mg

Exchange: 1 starch

For the icing per serving:

Calories	Protein	Carbohydrates	Fat	Sodium
56.11	1.78 g	9.86 g	0.94 g	19.17 mg

Exchange: 1½ starches; ½ milk

Spicy Applesauce Cake

Here is another moist and flavorful cake made with prune puree. For increased apple flavor, make the puree with apple juice rather than water. The cake is delicious served either plain or with several table-spoons of applesauce as a topping.

Nonstick cooking spray for the
  baking pan
2 cups all-purpose flour plus 1
  tablespoon for dusting the pan
½ cup Prune Puree (page 336)
3 tablespoons granulated sugar
  substitute
1 cup Applesauce (page 307) or
  unsweetened commercial
  applesauce

The equivalent of 2 eggs in egg
  substitute, beaten
1½ teaspoons baking soda
½ teaspoon salt
2 teaspoons ground cinnamon
½ teaspoon ground nutmeg
½ teaspoon ground ginger
½ cup raisins

Preheat the oven to 350°F. Coat a 9-by-13-inch baking pan with the nonstick cooking spray and dust with 1 tablespoon of the flour.

In a large bowl with an electric mixer, beat the prune puree and gradually add the sugar substitute and beat well. Add the applesauce and beat. Beat in the egg substitute and mix thoroughly.

Meanwhile, in another bowl, mix together the 2 cups of flour, the baking soda, salt, cinnamon, nutmeg, and ginger. Add this to the mixture in the mixing bowl and blend the dry mixture with the wet mixture until just combined.

With a spoon, stir in the raisins and spread the batter in the prepared pan. Bake for 35 to 40 minutes. The cake is done when a skewer inserted in the center of the cake comes out clean.

Cool the cake in the pan for about 5 minutes and then turn out onto a rack to cool. Cut into 3-by-3¼-inch pieces and serve. You may serve the cake with applesauce as a topping if you wish, or you may want to serve it plain.

YIELD: 1 cake (12 servings)   SERVING SIZE: 1 (3-by-3¼-inch) piece

Calories	Protein	Carbohydrates	Fat	Sodium
106	2 g	22 g	1 g	40 mg

Exchange: 1 starch; ½ fruit

Carrot Cake

This cake is quick and delicious and low in fat. When making the prune puree, use unsweetened natural apple juice instead of water.

Nonstick cooking spray for the
    baking pan
4 cups peeled and grated carrots,
    packed loosely
5 tablespoons granulated sugar
    substitute
1 cup drained crushed pineapple
    packed in natural juices with no
    sugar added
1 cup Prune Puree made with apple
    juice (page 336)

4 large egg whites
2½ teaspoons vanilla extract
2 cups all-purpose flour
2 teaspoons baking soda
1 teaspoon ground cinnamon
1 teaspoon ground nutmeg
½ teaspoon salt
¾ cup peeled, cored, and shredded
    apples (Granny Smith, Newton,
    or Pippin)

Preheat the oven to 375°F. Coat a 9-by-13-inch baking pan with the nonstick cooking spray.

In a large bowl, combine the carrots, sugar substitute, pineapple, prune puree, egg whites, and vanilla. Stir to blend thoroughly.

Add the flour, baking soda, cinnamon, nutmeg, and salt and mix so that all of the ingredients are thoroughly incorporated.

Gently stir in the shredded apples and pour the batter into the prepared baking pan. Bake for 40 to 45 minutes, until a skewer inserted in the center of the cake comes out clean.

Cool the pan on a rack and either remove the cake from the pan or leave it in the pan. Cut into 3-by-3¼-inch pieces and serve.

YIELD: 1 cake (12 servings)   SERVING SIZE: 1 (3-by-3¼-inch) piece

Calories	Protein	Carbohydrates	Fat	Sodium
109	3 g	24 g	0 g	194 mg

Exchange: 1 starch; ½ fruit

Creole Rice Custard

A custard is a heated sauce made from milk, eggs, and sugar, often flavored with vanilla or grated zest. It should never be boiled, merely simmered.

This dish is a nineteenth-century favorite and is a great dessert to use when you are serving a large group. I call it Creole because it is made with rice. The leftovers can be held in the refrigerator for 2 to 3 days. The recipe can easily be doubled or tripled.

½ cup long-grain white rice

1 cup cold water

½ teaspoon salt

½ teaspoon ground white pepper

½ teaspoon unsalted, low-fat margarine

1⅔ cups 1% or 2% milk

3 tablespoons fresh orange juice

The equivalent of 3 eggs in egg substitute, lightly beaten

¼ cup granulated sugar substitute

1 tablespoon finely grated orange zest

2 teaspoons finely grated lime or lemon zest

1 teaspoon vanilla extract

1 teaspoon ground nutmeg

Put the rice, cold water, salt, pepper, and margarine in a large (at least 3-quart), heavy-bottomed pot and bring to a boil over high heat.

Stir once with a large fork, reduce the heat to very low, and cover with a lid that fits tightly.

Cook for exactly 15 minutes without uncovering the pot, then remove the pot from the heat, uncover, and stir with a large fork to fluff the rice.

Return the pot to the heat, add the milk and orange juice, and bring slowly to a boil, stirring frequently.

Meanwhile, in a small bowl with a whisk, beat the egg substitute and sugar substitute together until the mixture is light and pale yellow. Add the orange zest and lime zest to the egg mixture and stir. Add the egg mixture to the simmering custard and cook over low heat for about 5 minutes. At this point the rice should be very soft and the mixture should begin to thicken. Add the vanilla and nutmeg to the pot, stirring to combine.

Remove the pot from the heat. Pour the custard into a shallow 8-by-8-inch baking dish and allow it to cool at room temperature.

Serve warm, or cover with plastic wrap, refrigerate, and serve chilled.

YIELD: 6 servings

SERVING SIZE: 1 (4-by-2⅔-inch) square

Calories	Protein	Carbohydrates	Fat	Sodium
131	7 g	17 g	0.83 g	126 mg

Exchange: 1 milk; ½ starch

Fresh Fruit Soufflé

This dish is quite simple to make, and you will find yourself making it again and again and enjoying it each and every time. I frequently make the soufflé with applesauce and it works especially well, but you can use fresh, frozen, or canned fruit. If you use canned fruit, make sure that it is completely drained, is unsweetened, and has no salt. If you use the frozen, use only IQF (individually quick-frozen) fruit with no added sugar or salt.

I have also used fresh fruit with great success, especially any fresh berry and apricots. If you use fresh apricots, you do need to peel them, but they do not need to be cooked. *All fruit must be thoroughly drained.* Puree the fruit in a blender, food processor, or food mill and blend, chop, or grind it until it has a fine consistency.

A soufflé should be served as soon as it comes out of the oven, and dessert soufflés are especially susceptible to falling. So pull the soufflé from the oven and serve immediately.

Nonstick cooking spray for the soufflé dish

A scant ½ teaspoon sugar to coat the soufflé dish

1 lime or lemon

¾ cup fresh or canned fruit puree or Applesauce (page 307)

Dash of salt

¼ teaspoon ground nutmeg (if using any fruit other than applesauce)

Dash of ground cardamom (if using any fruit other than applesauce)

1 to 2 tablespoons granulated sugar substitute

3 egg whites

Preheat the oven to 365°F. Lightly coat a 1-quart soufflé dish with the nonstick cooking spray and sprinkle it with the ½ teaspoon of sugar.

Grate the zest of the lime. Cut the lime in half and squeeze 1 tablespoon of the juice. Heat the fruit puree in a small pan over medium heat and add the lime zest, lime juice, salt, nutmeg and cardamom (if you don't use applesauce), and sugar substitute. Stir to blend and then remove the pot from the heat.

Beat the egg whites until they are pretty stiff, but not dry.

With a whisk, whip the egg whites into the hot puree, making sure that the mixture is thoroughly combined.

Spoon the mixture into the prepared soufflé dish and bake for 25 to 28 minutes.

Pull from the oven and serve immediately.

YIELD: 6 servings   SERVING SIZE: ½ cup

Calories	Protein	Carbohydrates	Fat	Sodium
39	2 g	7 g	0 g	38 mg

Exchange: ½ fruit

Rice Pudding

This pudding is made on top of the stove, much like tapioca pudding, and the consistency is much the same, very creamy. I like to serve it with warmed applesauce, but it is delicious on its own, either warm or cold.

5 tablespoons long-grain white
　rice
⅔ cup water
3 cups skim milk
¼ cup nonfat dry milk
1 cinnamon stick
5 tablespoons granulated sugar
　substitute

½ cup black currants, golden
　raisins, or raisins
1 egg or 3 tablespoons egg substitute
2 teaspoons vanilla extract
Applesauce (page 307), warmed for
　serving, optional
Ground nutmeg, ground allspice, or
　ground cinnamon to taste

Combine the rice and the water in a 3- or 4-quart saucepan and bring to a low boil over medium heat. Lower the heat and simmer the rice until all of the water is absorbed (about 7 to 8 minutes).

Add the skim milk and the nonfat dry milk to the rice, stirring to thoroughly combine.

Add the cinnamon stick and bring the mixture to a boil quickly over fairly high heat, then reduce the heat to a simmer, cover, and cook for 16 to 18 minutes.

Stir in the sugar substitute and the currants. Cook about 10 minutes more, until the pudding has a creamy consistency and the rice is tender.

Remove the saucepan from the heat. In a small bowl, whisk the egg with a little of the hot pudding. Add this mixture to the pudding in the pan, combining thoroughly. Return the pan to the heat, and while stirring constantly, heat the pudding until it starts to thicken.

Remove the pan from the heat and stir in the vanilla.

The pudding may be served either warm or cold. In either case, top with a few spoonfuls of the applesauce, if desired, and then sprinkle with the nutmeg, allspice, or cinnamon.

YIELD: 6 servings   SERVING SIZE: ½ cup

Calories	Protein	Carbohydrates	Fat	Sodium
133	7 g	23 g	1 g	92 mg

Exchange: ½ milk; 1 starch

Blueberry or Blackberry Pudding with Lemon Wine Sauce

This pudding is very quick and easy to put together and takes 30 to 45 minutes to bake. The lemon wine sauce is very quickly assembled as well and takes about 10 minutes to simmer. The pudding may be served either hot or cold with the sauce served warm. If you want the pudding to be cold, allow enough time for it to chill before serving, and make the sauce just before serving so that it will be warm.

¼ cup plus 1½ teaspoons all-purpose flour
1 teaspoon baking powder
4 tablespoons granulated sugar substitute
¼ teaspoon ground coriander
2 cups ripe blueberries or blackberries, thoroughly rinsed and drained

The equivalent of 1 egg in egg substitute, beaten
2 teaspoons melted low-fat margarine
Zest and juice of 1 large lemon or lime
¼ cup unsweetened natural apple juice
¼ cup dry red wine
1½ teaspoons low-fat margarine

Preheat the oven to 300°F.

Sift together ¼ cup of the flour, the baking powder, 2 tablespoons of the granulated sugar substitute, and the coriander and set aside.

Place the berries in a medium stainless steel or glass bowl and sprinkle the sifted mixture over them.

Combine the egg substitute and melted margarine and pour over the entire mixture. Gently mix the pudding, being careful not to mash the berries.

Place the mixture in an 8-inch round cake pan and bake for 30 to 45 minutes, until the pudding is thick and bubbly.

Meanwhile, in a small saucepan, whisk together the rest of the granulated sugar substitute, the remaining 1½ teaspoons of flour, the lemon zest and juice, apple juice, red wine, and margarine and bring the sauce to a boil. Turn down the heat to low and simmer the sauce for 12 to 15 minutes or until it is thick and opaque.

Spoon the pudding into individual serving dishes and top with the sauce.

YIELD: 2½ cups of pudding and ¾ to 1 cup of sauce

SERVING SIZE: ½ cup of pudding and 2 to 3 tablespoons of sauce

Calories	Protein	Carbohydrates	Fat	Sodium
100	2 g	15 g	3 g	96 mg

Exchange: 1 fruit

Sourdough Bread Pudding

This is a variation on an old favorite. Sourdough French bread is one of the few almost totally fat-free breads. It makes a dessert that is delicious whether served warm or cold. You need to cut the crusts off French bread, but if you cannot find French sourdough, you can use any white bread and not cut off the crusts.

After you have put the bread pudding together, refrigerate it for at least an hour or up to 3 hours before you bake it. The longer you are able to soak it, the "creamier" it will be. The baking dish has to be inserted into a larger dish with an inch of water surrounding it.

Nonstick cooking spray for the
   baking dish
1 cup evaporated skim milk
2 cups 1% milk
The equivalent of 3 eggs in egg
   substitute
¼ cup granulated sugar substitute
¼ teaspoon salt
½ cup raisins

1½ teaspoons vanilla extract
½ teaspoon ground cinnamon
½ teaspoon ground nutmeg
1 teaspoon grated lemon zest
6 thick slices day-old French
   sourdough bread with the crusts
   trimmed off, or 7 slices day-old
   white bread with the crusts left
   on, cut into cubes

Lightly coat a 2-quart baking dish with the nonstick cooking spray.

With a whisk, mix together thoroughly the evaporated skim milk, 1% milk, egg substitute, sugar substitute, salt, raisins, vanilla, cinnamon, nutmeg, and lemon zest. Pour this mixture over the bread cubes in a large bowl and toss and stir until the bread is absolutely saturated. To make sure that the bread is completely soaked, squeeze it with your hands.

Put the soaked bread and all of the milky liquid into the prepared baking dish and pat it down (do not pack it down) so that all of the bread is as wet as it can possibly be. Cover the dish with plastic wrap and refrigerate it for at least 1 hour.

Preheat the oven to 325°F.

Put the baking dish into a larger dish containing about 1 inch of hot water. Cover and bake for 30 minutes. Uncover and bake for 30 minutes more. The pudding is done when a knife inserted in the center comes out clean.

Serve warm or cold, with fruit or plain.

YIELD: 8 servings   SERVING SIZE: 1 (3-by-3-inch) square

Calories	Protein	Carbohydrates	Fat	Sodium
155	8 g	24 g	3 g	222 mg

Exchange: 1 milk; 1 starch

Lime and Coconut Mousse

This mousse, although it requires advance preparation, is light, delicious, and quite worth the effort. I give instructions for using a food processor, but it also can be made with an electric mixer. It does, however, take a bit more time. If you use an electric mixer, be sure to follow the descriptive instructions for the texture and the color. The final putting together of the mousse is done with a wire whisk whether you use a food processor in the initial steps or not.

The mousse can be made up to 2 weeks or so in advance and held in the freezer until you are ready to serve it. I would advise, at the very least, to prepare the mousse the day before, as it takes 1 hour for the coconut milk to rest before it can be used, 25 minutes for the mousse to sit in the refrigerator before adding the whipped topping, and then several hours for the mousse to freeze.

Do remember that on the day you wish to serve the mousse, you need to allow about 2½ hours for it to soften enough in the refrigerator to serve. You can put it in the refrigerator on the way to work and serve it that night. You can double the recipe if you so desire.

¾ cup 1% milk
¼ cup shredded unsweetened coconut (available at health food stores and specialty markets, and at many supermarkets)
4 medium limes

1½ teaspoons unflavored gelatin
The equivalent of 1½ eggs in egg substitute, lightly beaten
¼ cup granulated sugar substitute
½ cup nonfat, nondairy whipped topping

In a small, heavy-bottomed pan, heat the milk over medium heat, almost to a boil. Stir in the coconut and simmer for 1½ to 2 minutes. Remove the pan from the heat, cover, and let stand for 1 hour.

Strain the coconut milk through a fine-meshed strainer into a small bowl, pressing on the coconut meat itself with a large spoon to extract as much liquid as possible. Discard the coconut meat and set the milk aside.

Squeeze the juice of 3 of the limes to measure ⅓ cup. Pour the lime juice into a small bowl. Put about 2 cups of water in a small saucepan (large enough to accommodate the bowl into which you have put the lime juice) and bring the water to a simmer. This step is not necessary if you have a microwave.

Sprinkle the gelatin on top of the lime juice in the small bowl. Put the bowl into the small saucepan of simmering water and stir until the gelatin dissolves. Or you can put the small bowl in the microwave and "cook" on medium for 40 seconds.

Grate the zest from the remaining lime to measure 2 teaspoons. Cut the lime in half and squeeze 2 tablespoons of the juice. Set aside.

In a food processor, process the egg substitute and sugar substitute for 2 minutes. The mixture should be thick and light in color. With the machine running, pour in the 2 tablespoons of lime juice, the coconut milk, and the gelatin mixture and process for 10 seconds.

Pour the mixture into a bowl and refrigerate for about 25 minutes. You want the mixture to be thick but not quite set.

Take the bowl from the refrigerator and with a wire whisk, beat the mixture until it is smooth. Whisk in the lime zest. Spoon the whipped topping on top and whisk only until it is combined. Don't overbeat! Transfer the mousse either to individual serving cups or to a 3-cup serving dish and freeze until solid. Soften the mousse in the refrigerator for about 1 hour if you use the individual cups or 2 to 2½ hours if you use the large bowl. Serve.

YIELD: 3 cups   SERVING SIZE: ½ cup

Calories	Protein	Carbohydrates	Fat	Sodium
96	3 g	5 g	8 g	38 mg

Exchange: ½ milk; 1 fat

Orange, Grapefruit, and Raspberry Terrine

This terrine is fast and easy to make, but it requires freezing overnight before it can be served. It is a dish that is spectacular in its presentation and has the added advantage of being made with fruits that are easily available and inexpensive in the winter. I like to use it at brunch as well as at dinner.

Whether I use it as a dessert item or a brunch item, I like to serve it with a raspberry sauce that is made by blending about ½ cup of thawed frozen raspberries (with no additives) in a blender with a dash of lime juice and a scant teaspoon of granulated sugar. Spoon a few tablespoons of the sauce on a small serving plate and then place the slice of terrine at an angle on the sauce (so that the sauce shows on the plate after you have placed the terrine on it). The sauce is optional, however, and the terrine is very tasty without it. I put ½ cup of raspberries in the terrine whether or not I make the sauce.

On the day you serve the terrine, allow about 30 minutes for it to defrost before serving. You want it to be cold, not frozen. The terrine may be kept in the refrigerator for several days after you first serve it.

3 large navel or Valencia oranges
(use navels from fall to spring
and Valencias from spring to
fall)
2 mandarin oranges
3 large Texas Ruby Red grapefruits
(if not available, ripe pink
grapefruits will do)
2 large limes or lemons
½ cup frozen raspberries with no
additives

Fresh orange juice if needed to make
the 3 cups of juice for the terrine
2 envelopes (or 1½ tablespoons)
unflavored gelatin
5 tablespoons granulated sugar
substitute
Raspberry sauce (see headnote),
optional
Fresh mint leaves for garnish,
optional

On the day before you wish to serve the terrine, line a 9-by-5-inch loaf pan with a large piece of plastic wrap. Be sure that the plastic wrap hangs over the sides of the pan at least 4 inches.

At this point, using a zester or a grater with small holes, rub the rind of the oranges until you have 4 teaspoons of zest. Set aside.

Cut the ends off the oranges, grapefruits, and limes. Stand a fruit on one of its cut ends, and with a very sharp paring knife, carefully cut away the peel, being sure to remove every bit of the white pith. Repeat this procedure until each piece of fruit is peeled.

Holding the peeled citrus in one hand and with the paring knife in the other, cut out the sections of fruit in one curving motion. Do this over a bowl so that you can save the juices. As you are doing this procedure, be sure that you are cutting out the section of fruit only, leaving behind the membrane that holds the fruit section attached to the core. Do this with all of the oranges, grapefruits, and limes. Check to make sure that there are no seeds. Squeeze the juice from the citrus cores and membranes into the small bowl over which you have cut the fruit.

After you have drained and saved all of the juice from the fruit, toss the oranges, grapefruits, and limes and put a 3-inch layer of this mixture in the loaf pan. Follow with a layer of the frozen raspberries and then cover that layer with the remainder of the citrus mixture. Set aside.

Measure the juice mixture that you have gleaned from the fruit, making sure that you have 3 cups. Use the fresh juice that you have held on the side if needed to make the 3 cups. Put this juice in a small saucepan. Of these 3 cups, take out 6 tablespoons and put it in another small saucepan or in a small microwavable dish with the 4 teaspoons of orange zest that have been held on the side. If you don't have a microwave, quickly bring the juice and the zest to a boil and cook it for about 2 minutes. If you do have a microwave, put the mixture in, cover loosely with plastic wrap, and on high, microwave for about 20 seconds. Whichever method you use, after quickly boiling the mixture, set it aside to cool.

Stir the gelatin into the cooled juice and zest and again set aside to let the gelatin soften.

Add the granulated sugar substitute to the remaining juice in the small saucepan, bring to a boil, then simmer for about 10 to 12 minutes, at which point the volume of the juice should be reduced by about one-third. Stir in the softened gelatin mixture immediately, stirring until it is dissolved.

Pour the juice mixture over the fruits already layered in the pan and wrap the excess plastic wrap over the top of the terrine. Freeze the terrine overnight.

When you are ready to serve, put the pan into a larger one that you have filled with very warm water. Remove the terrine pan from the other pan after about 30 seconds in the water. Unwrap the plastic wrap from the top and shake it a bit to loosen the terrine in the pan. Lift the terrine from the pan and turn it upside down onto a flat cutting surface. Dispose of the plastic wrap and cut the terrine into ¾-inch slices and put them (not overlapping) on a platter to defrost.

Put the raspberry sauce on a plate and, lifting the slice of terrine with a serving spatula, arrange the slice on the sauce at an angle, garnish with the mint leaves, if desired, and serve.

YIELD: 1 (9-by-5-inch) terrine   SERVING SIZE: 1 (¾-inch) slice
(12 servings)

Calories	Protein	Carbohydrates	Fat	Sodium
58	1 g	14 g	0 g	0 mg

Exchange: 1 fruit

Chocolate Crepes

Once again unsweetened cocoa powder has put the skinny on chocolate. It has only 115 calories per ounce (⅓ cup) and has very little cocoa butter, which is what puts the saturated fat into chocolate. This chocolate crepe recipe uses unsweetened cocoa and egg substitute, which lowers both the fat amount and the cholesterol amount, so it's perfect for our purposes.

The easiest way to prepare these crepes is to make them the night before, along with the filling you plan to use, so that all you have to do is just fill them when you are ready to serve.

You can hold them in the refrigerator for several days or put them in freezer bags and freeze them until you are ready to use them. In the freezer, they hold beautifully for several months.

The equivalent of 2 eggs in egg
    substitute
1 cup lukewarm water
1 cup lukewarm unsweetened
    natural apple juice
2 cups all-purpose flour
¼ cup unsweetened cocoa powder
2 tablespoons granulated sugar
    substitute

½ teaspoon salt
1½ teaspoons vanilla extract
Nonstick cooking spray for the crepe
    pan
Fresh fruit, Spicy Apple Slices
    (page 308), Vanilla Custard
    Cream (page 363), or Fruit
    Compote (page 312) to fill the
    crepes

In a medium bowl, beat the egg substitute. Whisk in the water, apple juice, flour, cocoa powder, sugar substitute, salt, and vanilla.

Heat a crepe pan or an 8-inch nonstick skillet over medium heat and lightly coat it with the nonstick cooking spray. When the pan is hot, add a scant ¼ cup of the crepe batter, holding the pan up and tilting it so that the batter coats the bottom of the pan in a thin layer.

Cook the crepe for several minutes, until the edges start to come up from the bottom of the pan. Flip the crepe over with a rubber spatula and let it cook for 20 to 30 seconds. Turn the crepe out onto a clean dish towel and while it is cooling, continue cooking until all of the batter is used. Coat with the cooking spray as it becomes necessary.

If you cook the crepes to use the next day (see headnote), layer them between sheets of waxed paper and either store them in an airtight container or wrap them very tightly in plastic wrap and refrigerate until you are ready to use them.

Fill the crepes with the filling of your choice and serve.

YIELD: 16 to 18 crepes　　　　　　　SERVING SIZE: 1 crepe

Calories	Protein	Carbohydrates	Fat	Sodium
66	2 g	12 g	0 g	29 mg

Exchange: 1 starch

Cream Puffs

This is based on a tried-and-true recipe that my mother has used for years and years. And, I must add, it has taken me about that long to get it. She uses this recipe for both cream puffs and eclairs. I prefer to make cream puffs because they are smaller and make a beautiful presentation whether served on a silver tray or a pottery plate. I usually fill them with just the plain Vanilla Custard Cream filling, but I have combined chopped fresh fruit with nonfat, nondairy whipped topping and stuffed the cream puffs and found them to be delicious. You'll want to try both. I don't use egg substitute in making cream puffs, as it simply does not work. Use low-cholesterol eggs instead.

There is one real trick to baking the cream puffs. You cannot open the oven door after you put the puffs in until they are done. It's simple: don't open the door, because if you do, they will fall flatter than a tortilla.

Nonstick cooking spray for the
   cookie sheets
1 cup all-purpose flour
½ teaspoon salt
1 stick (½ cup) low-fat margarine

1 cup boiling water
4 (low-cholesterol) eggs
Vanilla Custard Cream
   (page 363)
Confectioners' sugar
   substitute

Preheat the oven to 400°F. Coat 2 cookie sheets with the nonstick cooking spray.

Sift the flour and measure out 1 cup. Place the cup of flour and the salt in a small bowl.

Combine the margarine and the boiling water in a medium saucepan over high heat and stir until the margarine is melted.

Immediately turn the heat down low, add the flour mixture, and stir very vigorously until the mixture leaves the sides of the pan in a smooth, compact ball.

Remove the pan from the heat and add the eggs, one at a time, beating the mixture with a large spoon after each addition. The mixture must have a "satinlike" sheen.

Drop by the tablespoonful 1 inch apart onto the prepared cookie sheets, shaping into mounds that point up in the center (like a pyramid).

Bake for 35 minutes. Do not open the oven door during the baking process, as the cream puffs will fall.

Remove the pans from the oven, slice the tops off the puffs, and scoop out the centers. Cool completely on a rack. Using a teaspoon, fill with vanilla custard cream, and dust lightly with confectioners' sugar substitute.

YIELD: 44 small cream puffs   SERVING SIZE: 2 puffs

Calories	Protein	Carbohydrates	Fat	Sodium
46	1 g	4 g	3 g	73 mg

Exchange: ¼ starch; ½ fat

Vanilla Custard Cream

Quick and easy, this recipe works well as a custard sauce, a filling for dessert crepes, and, of course, as a filling for Cream Puffs (page 361).

The only labor-intensive aspect of this custard is that it *must* be stirred with a whisk the entire time you are cooking it or you will end up with a scrambled egg–like mixture, which is definitely not what you want.

2 cups 1% milk

¼ cup granulated sugar substitute

Dash of salt

½ cup all-purpose flour

The equivalent of 2 eggs in egg substitute, beaten

1 teaspoon vanilla extract

Heat the milk in a medium, heavy-bottomed saucepan over medium heat.

Meanwhile, whisk together the sugar substitute, salt, flour, and egg substitute.

Add the egg mixture to the heated milk, whisking all the while.

Cook over medium heat until the mixture becomes thick, being sure to whisk the whole time you are cooking. It does not take long for the mixture to thicken.

When the custard is thick enough to coat a spoon, remove the saucepan from the heat and allow the custard to cool. When it is cool, stir in the vanilla.

YIELD: 2½ cups   SERVING SIZE: 2⅓ teaspoons
                                  per puff or crepe

Calories	Protein	Carbohydrates	Fat	Sodium
8	0 g	1 g	0 g	6 mg

Exchange: Free

Exchange Lists

The following exchange lists are given here by permission of the American Diabetes Association.

T he reason for dividing food into six different groups is that foods vary in their carbohydrate, protein, fat, and calorie content. Each exchange list contains foods that are alike — each choice contains about the same amount of carbohydrates, protein, fat, and calories.

The following chart shows the amount of these nutrients in one serving from each exchange list.

Exchange List	Carbohydrates (g)	Protein (g)	Fat (g)	Calories
Starch/Bread	15	3	trace	80
Meat				
Lean	—	7	3	55
Medium-Fat	—	7	5	75
High-Fat	—	7	8	100
Vegetable	5	2	—	25
Fruit	15	—	—	60
Milk				
Skim	12	8	trace	90
Low-fat	12	8	5	120
Whole	12	8	8	150
Fat	—	—	5	45

As you read the exchange lists, you will notice that one choice often is a larger amount of food than another choice from the same list. Because foods are so different, each food is measured or weighed so the amount of carbohydrate, protein, fat, and calories is the same in each choice.

You will notice symbols on some foods in the exchange groups. Foods that are high in fiber (3 grams or more per exchange) have a 🌾 (fiber) symbol. High-fiber foods are good for you. It is important to eat more of these foods.

Foods that are high in sodium (400 milligrams or more of sodium per exchange) have a 🥄 (salt) symbol; foods that have 400 milligrams or more of sodium if two or more exchanges are eaten have a ★ (star) symbol. It's a good idea to limit your intake of high-salt foods, especially if you have high blood pressure.

If you have a favorite food that is not included in any of these groups, ask your dietitian about it. That food can probably be worked into your meal plan, at least now and then.

Starch/Bread List

Each item in this list contains approximately 15 grams of carbohydrates, 3 grams of protein, a trace of fat, and 80 calories. Whole grain products average about 2 grams of fiber per exchange. Some foods are higher in fiber. Those foods that contain 3 or more grams of fiber per exchange are identified with the fiber symbol 🌾.

You can choose your starch exchanges from any of the items on this list. If you want to eat a starch food that is not on this list, the general rule is that:

- ½ cup of cereal, grain, or pasta is one exchange
- 1 ounce of a bread product is one exchange

Your dietitian can help you be more exact.

CEREALS/GRAINS/PASTA

🌾 Bran cereals, concentrated (such as Bran Buds, All-Bran)	⅓ cup
🌾 Bran cereals, flaked	½ cup
Bulgur (cooked)	½ cup
Cooked cereals	½ cup
Cornmeal (dry)	2½ tbsp.
Grape-Nuts	3 tbsp.
Grits (cooked)	½ cup
Other ready-to-eat unsweetened cereals	¾ cup
Pasta (cooked)	½ cup

🌾 3 grams or more of fiber per exchange

Puffed cereal	1½ cups
Rice, white or brown (cooked)	⅓ cup
Shredded wheat	½ cup
❧ Wheat germ	3 tbsp.

DRIED BEANS/PEAS/LENTILS

❧ Beans and peas (cooked) (such as kidney, white, split, black-eyed)	⅓ cup
❧ Lentils (cooked)	⅓ cup
❧ Baked beans	¼ cup

STARCHY VEGETABLES

❧ Corn	½ cup
❧ Corn on cob, 6 in. long	1
❧ Lima beans	½ cup
❧ Peas, green (canned or frozen)	½ cup
❧ Plantain	½ cup
Potato, baked	1 small (3 oz.)
Potato, mashed	½ cup
❧ Squash, winter (acorn, butternut)	1 cup
Yam, sweet potato, plain	⅓ cup

BREAD

Bagel	½ (1 oz.)
Bread sticks, crisp, 4 in. long by ½ in.	2 (⅔ oz.)
Croutons, low-fat	1 cup

❧3 grams or more of fiber per exchange

English muffin	½
Frankfurter or hamburger bun	½ (1 oz.)
Pita, 6 in. across	½
Plain roll, small	1 (1 oz.)
Raisin, unfrosted	1 slice (1 oz.)
Rye, pumpernickel	1 slice (1 oz.)
Tortilla, 6 in. across	1
White (including French, Italian)	1 slice (1 oz.)
Whole wheat	1 slice (1 oz.)

CRACKERS/SNACKS

Animal crackers	8
Graham crackers, 2½ in. square	3
Matzoh	¾ oz.
Melba toast	5 slices
Oyster crackers	24
Popcorn (popped, no fat added)	3 cups
Pretzels	¾ oz.
❧ Rye crisp, 2 in. by 3½ in.	4
Saltine-type crackers	6
❧ Whole wheat crackers, no fat added (crisp breads, such as Finn, Kavli, Wasa)	2–4 slices (¾ oz.)

STARCH FOODS PREPARED WITH FAT

(Count as 1 starch/bread exchange, plus 1 fat exchange.)

Biscuit, 2½ in. across	1
Chow mein noodles	½ cup

❧3 grams or more of fiber per exchange

Corn bread, 2-in. cube	1 (2 oz.)
Cracker, round butter type	6
French-fried potatoes, 2 in. to 3½ in. long	10 (1½ oz.)
Muffin, plain, small	1
Pancake, 4 in. across	2
Stuffing, bread (prepared)	¼ cup
Taco shell, 6 in. across	2
Waffle, 4½ in. square	1
❧ Whole wheat crackers, fat added (such as Triscuit)	4–6 (1 oz.)

Meat List

Each serving of meat and substitutes on this list contains about 7 grams of protein. The amount of fat and number of calories varies, depending on what kind of meat or substitute you choose. The list is divided into three parts based on the amount of fat and calories: lean meat, medium-fat meat, and high-fat meat. One ounce (one meat exchange) of each of these includes:

	Carbohydrates (g)	Protein (g)	Fat (g)	Calories
Lean	0	7	3	55
Medium-Fat	0	7	5	75
High-Fat	0	7	8	100

❧ 3 grams or more of fiber per exchange

You are encouraged to use more lean and medium-fat meat, poultry, and fish in your meal plan. This will help decrease your fat intake, which may help decrease your risk for heart disease. The items from the high-fat group are high in saturated fat, cholesterol, and calories. You should limit your choices from the high-fat group to three times per week. Meat and substitutes do not contribute any fiber to your meal plan.

TIPS

1. Bake, roast, broil, grill, or boil these foods rather than frying them with added fat.
2. Use a nonstick pan spray or a nonstick pan to brown or fry these foods.
3. Trim off visible fat before and after cooking.
4. Do not add flour, bread crumbs, coating mixes, or fat to these foods when preparing them.
5. Weigh meat after removing bones and fat, and after cooking. Three ounces of cooked meat is about equal to 4 ounces of raw meat. Some examples of meat portions are:

   2 ounces meat (2 meat exchanges) =
      1 small chicken leg or thigh
      ½ cup cottage cheese or tuna

   3 ounces meat (3 meat exchanges) =
      1 medium pork chop
      1 small hamburger
      ½ of a whole chicken breast
      1 unbreaded fish fillet
      cooked meat, about the size of a deck of cards

6. Restaurants usually serve prime cuts of meat, which are high in fat and calories.

LEAN MEAT AND SUBSTITUTES
(One exchange is equal to any one of the following items.)

BEEF: *USDA Select or Choice grades of lean beef,* 1 oz.
such as round, sirloin, and flank steak;
tenderloin; and chipped beef 🥩

PORK: *Lean pork, such as fresh ham; canned,* 1 oz.
cured, or boiled ham 🥩*; Canadian bacon*
🥩*; tenderloin*

VEAL: *All cuts are lean except for veal cutlets* 1 oz.
(ground or cubed). Examples of lean veal
are chops and roasts

POULTRY: *Chicken, turkey, Cornish hen (without*
skin) 1 oz.

FISH: *All fresh and frozen fish* 1 oz.
Crab, lobster, scallops, shrimp, clams 2 oz.
(fresh or canned in water)
Oysters 6 medium
Tuna ★ (canned in water) ¼ cup
Herring ★ (uncreamed or smoked) 1 oz.
Sardines (canned) 2 medium

WILD GAME: *Venison, rabbit, squirrel* 1 oz.
Pheasant, duck, goose (without skin) 1 oz.

CHEESE: *Any cottage cheese ★* ¼ cup
Grated Parmesan 2 tbsp.
Diet cheeses 🥩 *(with less than 55 calories* 1 oz.
per ounce)

OTHER: *95% fat-free luncheon meat* 🥩 1½ oz.
Egg whites 3 whites
Egg substitutes with less than 55 calories ½ cup
per ½ cup

🥩 400 mg or more of sodium per exchange
★ 400 mg or more of sodium if two or more exchanges are eaten

MEDIUM-FAT MEAT AND SUBSTITUTES

(One exchange is equal to any one of the following items.)

BEEF:	*Most beef products fall into this category. Examples are: all ground beef, roast (rib, chuck, rump), steak (cubed, Porterhouse, T-bone), and meatloaf*	1 oz.
PORK:	*Most pork products fall into this category. Examples are: chops, loin roast, Boston butt, cutlets*	1 oz.
LAMB:	*Most lamb products fall into this category. Examples are: chops, leg, and roast*	1 oz.
VEAL:	*Cutlet (ground or cubed, unbreaded)*	1 oz.
POULTRY:	*Chicken (with skin), domestic duck or goose (well drained of fat), ground turkey*	1 oz.
FISH:	*Tuna ★ (canned in oil and drained)*	¼ cup
	Salmon ★ (canned)	¼ cup
CHEESE:	*Skim or part-skim milk cheeses, such as:*	
	Ricotta	¼ cup
	Mozzarella	1 oz.
	Diet cheeses 🥄 (with 56–80 calories per ounce)	1 oz.
OTHER:	*86% fat-free luncheon meat ★*	1 oz.
	Egg (high in cholesterol, limit to 3 per week)	1
	Egg substitutes with 56–80 calories per ¼ cup	¼ cup
	Tofu (2½ in. by 2¾ in. by 1 in.)	4 oz.
	Liver, heart, kidney, sweetbreads (high in cholesterol)	1 oz.

🥄 400 mg or more of sodium per exchange
★ 400 mg or more of sodium if two or more exchanges are eaten

HIGH-FAT MEAT AND SUBSTITUTES

Remember, these items are high in saturated fat, cholesterol, and calories, and should be used only three times per week.

(One exchange is equal to any one of the following items.)

BEEF:	*Most USDA Prime cuts of beef, such as ribs, corned beef* ★	1 oz.
PORK:	*Spareribs, ground pork, pork sausage* 🖋 *(patty or link)*	1 oz.
LAMB:	*Patties (ground lamb)*	1 oz.
FISH:	*Any fried fish product*	1 oz.
CHEESE:	*All regular cheeses, such as American* 🖋, *Blue* 🖋, *Cheddar* ★, *Monterey Jack* ★, *Swiss*	1 oz.
OTHER:	*Luncheon meat* 🖋, *such as bologna, salami, pimento loaf*	1 oz.
	Sausage 🖋, *such as Polish, Italian smoked*	1 oz.
	Knockwurst 🖋	1 oz.
	Bratwurst ★	1 oz.
	Frankfurter 🖋 *(turkey or chicken)*	1 frank (10/lb.)
	Peanut butter (contains unsaturated fat)	1 tbsp.

Count as one high-fat meat plus one fat exchange:

Frankfurter 🖋 *(beef, pork, or combination)*	1 frank (10/lb.)

🖋 400 mg or more of sodium per exchange
★ 400 mg or more of sodium if two or more exchanges are eaten

Vegetable List

Each vegetable serving on this list contains about 5 grams of carbohydrates, 2 grams of protein, and 25 calories. Vegetables contain 2–3 grams of dietary fiber. Vegetables that contain 400 mg or more of sodium per exchange are identified with a 🥖 symbol.

Vegetables are a good source of vitamins and minerals. Fresh and frozen vegetables have more vitamins and less added salt. Rinsing canned vegetables will remove much of the salt.

Unless otherwise noted, the serving size for vegetables (one vegetable exchange) is:

½ cup of cooked vegetables or vegetable juice

1 cup of raw vegetables

Artichoke (½ medium)

Asparagus

Beans (green, wax, Italian)

Bean sprouts

Beets

Broccoli

Brussels sprouts

Cabbage, cooked

Carrots

Cauliflower

Eggplant

Greens (collard, mustard, turnip)

Kohlrabi

Leeks

Mushrooms, cooked

Okra

Onions

Pea pods

Peppers (green)

Rutabaga

Sauerkraut 🥖

Spinach, cooked

Summer squash (crookneck)

Tomato (one large)

Tomato/vegetable juice 🥖

Turnips

Water chestnuts

Zucchini, cooked

Starchy vegetables such as corn, peas, and potatoes are found on the Starch/Bread List, page 367.

For free vegetables, see Free Foods List on page 382.

🥖 400 mg or more of sodium per exchange

Fruit List

Each item on this list contains about 15 grams of carbohydrates and 60 calories. Fresh, frozen, and dried fruits have about 2 grams of fiber per exchange. Fruits that have 3 or more grams of fiber per exchange have a 🌾 symbol. Fruit juices contain very little dietary fiber.

The carbohydrate and calorie content for a fruit exchange are based on the usual serving of the most commonly eaten fruits. Use fresh fruits or fruits frozen or canned without sugar added. Whole fruit is more filling than fruit juice and may be a better choice for those who are trying to lose weight. Unless otherwise noted, the serving size for one fruit exchange is:

½ cup of fresh fruit or fruit juice

¼ cup of dried fruit

FRESH, FROZEN, AND UNSWEETENED CANNED FRUIT

Apple (raw, 2 in. across)	1 apple
Applesauce (unsweetened)	½ cup
Apricots (medium, raw)	4 apricots
Apricots (canned)	½ cup, or 4 halves
Banana (9 in. long)	½ banana
🌾 Blackberries (raw)	¾ cup
🌾 Blueberries (raw)	¾ cup
Cantaloupe (5 in. across)	⅓ melon
(cubes)	1 cup
Cherries (large, raw)	12 cherries

🌾 3 or more grams of fiber per exchange

Cherries (canned)	½ cup
Figs (raw, 2 in. across)	2 figs
Fruit cocktail (canned)	½ cup
Grapefruit (medium)	½ grapefruit
Grapefruit (segments)	¾ cup
Grapes (small)	15 grapes
Honeydew melon (medium)	⅛ melon
(cubes)	1 cup
Kiwi (large)	1 kiwi
Mandarin oranges	¾ cup
Mango (small)	½ mango
❦ Nectarine (2½ in. across)	1 nectarine
Orange (2½ in. across)	1 orange
Papaya	1 cup
Peach (2¾ in. across)	1 peach, or ¾ cup
Peaches (canned)	½ cup or 2 halves
Pear	½ large, or 1 small
Pears (canned)	½ cup, or 2 halves
Persimmon (medium, native)	2 persimmons
Pineapple (raw)	¾ cup
Pineapple (canned)	⅓ cup
Plum (raw, 2 in. across)	2 plums
❦ Pomegranate	½ pomegranate
❦ Raspberries (raw)	1 cup
❦ Strawberries (raw, whole)	1¼ cup

❦ 3 or more grams of fiber per exchange

🌿 Tangerine (2½ in. across)   2 tangerines
   Watermelon (cubes)   1¼ cup

DRIED FRUIT

🌿 Apples   4 rings
🌿 Apricots   7 halves
   Dates   2½ medium
🌿 Figs   1½
🌿 Prunes   3 medium
   Raisins   2 tbsp.

FRUIT JUICE

Apple juice/cider   ½ cup
Cranberry juice cocktail ⅓ cup
Grapefruit juice   ½ cup
Grape juice   ⅓ cup
Orange juice   ½ cup
Pineapple juice   ½ cup
Prune juice   ⅓ cup

Milk List

Each serving of milk or milk products on this list contains about 12 grams of carbohydrates and 8 grams of protein. The amount of fat in milk is measured in percent (%) of butterfat. The calories vary, depending on what kind of milk you choose. The list is divided into three parts based on the amount of fat and calories: skim/very low-fat

🌿 3 or more grams of fiber per exchange

milk, low-fat milk, and whole milk. One serving (one milk exchange) of each of these includes:

	Carbohydrates (g)	Protein (g)	Fat (g)	Calories
Skim/Very Low-fat	12	8	trace	90
Low-fat	12	8	5	120
Whole	12	8	8	150

Milk is the body's main source of calcium, the mineral needed for growth and repair of bones. Yogurt is also a good source of calcium. Yogurt and many dry or powdered milk products have different amounts of fat. If you have questions about a particular item, read the label to find out the fat and calorie content.

Milk is good to drink, but it can also be added to cereal, and to other foods. Many tasty dishes such as sugar-free pudding are made with milk. Add life to plain yogurt by adding one of your fruit exchanges to it.

SKIM AND VERY LOW-FAT MILK

Skim milk	1 cup
½% milk	1 cup
1% milk	1 cup
Low-fat buttermilk	1 cup
Evaporated skim milk	½ cup
Dry nonfat milk	⅓ cup
Plain nonfat yogurt	8 oz.

LOW-FAT MILK

2% milk	1 cup
Plain low-fat yogurt (with added nonfat milk solids)	8 oz.

WHOLE MILK

The whole milk group has much more fat per serving than the skim and low-fat groups. Whole milk has more than 3¼% butterfat. Try to limit your choices from the whole milk group as much as possible.

Whole milk	1 cup
Evaporated whole milk	½ cup
Whole plain yogurt	8 oz.

Fat List

Each serving on the fat list contains about 5 grams of fat and 45 calories.

The foods on the fat list contain mostly fat, although some items may also contain a small amount of protein. All fats are high in calories and should be carefully measured. Everyone should modify fat intake by eating unsaturated fats instead of saturated fats. The sodium content of these foods varies widely. Check the label for sodium information.

UNSATURATED FATS

Avocado	⅛ medium
Margarine	1 tsp.
★Margarine, diet	1 tbsp.
Mayonnaise	1 tsp.
★Mayonnaise, reduced-calorie	1 tbsp.
Nuts and Seeds	
almonds, dry roasted	6 whole
cashews, dry roasted	1 tbsp.
pecans	2 whole
peanuts	20 small or 10 large
walnuts	2 whole
other nuts	1 tbsp.
seeds, pine nuts, sunflower (without shells)	1 tbsp.
pumpkin seeds	2 tsp.
Oil (corn, cottonseed, safflower, soybean, sunflower, olive, peanut)	1 tsp.
★Olives	10 small or 5 large
Salad dressing, mayonnaise-type	2 tsp.
Salad dressing, mayonnaise-type, reduced-calorie	1 tbsp.
★Salad dressing (oil varieties)	1 tbsp.
✒Salad dressing, reduced-calorie	2 tbsp.

(Two tablespoons of low-calorie salad dressing is a free food.)

✒ 400 mg or more of sodium per exchange
★ 400 mg or more of sodium if two or more exchanges are eaten

SATURATED FATS

Butter	1 tsp.
★Bacon	1 slice
Chitterlings	½ ounce
Coconut, shredded	2 tbsp.
Coffee whitener, liquid	2 tbsp.
Coffee whitener, powder	4 tsp.
Cream (light, coffee, table)	2 tbsp.
Cream, sour	2 tbsp.
Cream (heavy, whipping)	1 tbsp.
Cream cheese	1 tbsp.
★Salt pork	¼ ounce

Free Foods List

A free food is any food or drink that contains less than 20 calories per serving. You can eat as much as you want of those items that have no serving size specified. You may eat two or three servings per day of those items that have a specific serving size. Be sure to spread them out through the day.

DRINKS

Bouillon 🎀 or broth without fat
Bouillon, low-sodium
Carbonated drinks, sugar-free
Carbonated water
Club soda

Cocoa powder, unsweetened
(1 tbsp.)
Coffee/Tea
Drink mixes, sugar-free
Tonic water, sugar-free

🎀 400 mg or more of sodium per exchange
★ 400 mg or more of sodium if two or more exchanges are eaten

NONSTICK PAN SPRAY

FRUIT

Cranberries, unsweetened (½ cup)   Rhubarb, unsweetened (½ cup)

VEGETABLES

(raw, 1 cup)

Cabbage   Hot peppers
Celery   Mushrooms
Chinese cabbage 🌿   Radishes
Cucumber   Zucchini 🌿
Green onion

SALAD GREENS

Endive   Romaine
Escarole   Spinach
Lettuce

SWEET SUBSTITUTES

Candy, hard, sugar-free   Pancake syrup, sugar-free (1–
Gelatin, sugar-free   2 tbsp.)
Gum, sugar-free   Sugar substitutes (saccharin,
Jam/jelly, sugar-free (less than   aspartame)
    20 cal./2 tsp.)   Whipped topping (2 tbsp.)

🌿 3 grams or more of fiber per exchange

CONDIMENTS

Catsup (1 tbsp.)

Horseradish

Mustard

Pickles 🗡, dill, unsweetened

Salad dressing, low-calorie (2 tbsp.)

Taco sauce (3 tbsp.)

Vinegar

Seasonings can be very helpful in making food taste better. Be careful of how much sodium you use. Read the label, and choose those seasonings that do not contain sodium or salt.

Basil (fresh)

Celery seeds

Chili powder

Chives

Cinnamon

Curry

Dill

Flavoring extracts (vanilla, almond, walnut, peppermint, butter, lemon, etc.)

Garlic

Garlic powder

Herbs

Hot pepper sauce

Lemon

Lemon juice

Lemon pepper

Lime

Lime juice

Mint

Onion powder

Oregano

Paprika

Pepper

Pimento

Spices

Soy sauce 🗡

Soy sauce 🗡, low-sodium ("lite")

Wine, used in cooking (¼ cup)

Worcestershire sauce

🗡 400 mg or more of sodium per exchange

Foods for Occasional Use

Moderate amounts of some foods can be used in your meal plan in spite of their sugar or fat content, as long as you can maintain blood glucose control. The following list includes average exchange values for some of these foods. Because they are concentrated sources of carbohydrate, you will notice that the portion sizes are very small. Check with your dietitian for advice on how often and when you can eat them.

Food	Amount	Exchanges
Angel food cake	1/12 cake	2 starch
Cake, no icing	1/12 cake, or a 3-in. square	2 starch, 2 fat
Cookies	2 small (1¾ in. across)	1 starch, 1 fat
Frozen fruit yogurt	1/3 cup	1 starch
Gingersnaps	3	1 starch
Granola	1/4 cup	1 starch, 1 fat
Granola bars	1 small	1 starch, 1 fat
Ice cream, any flavor	1/2 cup	1 starch, 2 fat
Ice milk, any flavor	1/2 cup	1 starch, 1 fat
Sherbet, any flavor	1/4 cup	1 starch
Snack chips ★, all varieties	1 oz.	1 starch, 2 fat
Vanilla wafers	6 small	1 starch

★ 400 mg or more of sodium if two or more exchanges are eaten

Raw Shellfish Warning

The summer 1993 issue of *Professional Section News* of the American Diabetes Association published the following FDA warning concerning raw shellfish:

Patients with diabetes are among the population group that are at serious risk of Vibrio infection from eating raw shellfish. While it is not a threat to most healthy patients, certain susceptible patients can be exposed to the infection by eating raw or undercooked molluscan shellfish such as oysters, mussels, clams, and whole scallops. The population groups that are particularly vulnerable to severe illness, or even death, if they ingest contaminated seafood are those with liver disease, diabetes mellitus, immune disorders, and gastrointestinal disorders.

The high-risk season for raw shellfish consumption begins in April when warmer water encourages the growth of the bacteria Vibrio vulnificus. The symptoms of the infection include fever, chills, nausea, vomiting, and abdominal pain. The bacteria are killed when the shellfish are thoroughly cooked.

More information is available in a series of four brochures entitled "Get Hooked on Seafood Safety." For a free copy of the diabetes mellitus brochure, write to: FDA, Seafood Brochures, HFI40, 5600 Fishers Lane, Rockville, MD 20857. Be sure to specify you want the diabetes brochure.

This warning should be sufficient to stop you from eating raw or inadequately cooked shellfish or seafood of any kind. In my opinion, due to the special vulnerability of diabetics to inborn bacterial infection, all the food we eat should be thoroughly cooked. It is no longer considered safe to consume raw or even lightly cooked eggs, steak tartare, or other cuts of meat that are poorly or inadequately cooked.

Selected Reading List

BOOKS DEALING WITH THE DIABETIC DIET

The All-New Cookbook for Diabetics and Their Families, Oxmore House, 1989.

American Diabetes Association and American Dietetic Association. *The American Diabetes Association/The American Dietetic Association Family Cookbook,* vol. 2, Prentice Hall, 1984.

_____. *The American Diabetes Association/The American Dietetic Association Family Cookbook with Microwave Adaptations,* vol. 3, 1st ed., Prentice Hall, 1978.

_____. *American Dietetic Association Family Cookbook,* vols. 1 and 2, American Diabetes Association, 1986.

Blanchard, Pat. *Basic Menus and Recipes for Diabetics,* Creole Publishing, 1989.

Bowens, Angela. *The Diabetic Gourmet,* Harper & Row, 1981.

Budd, Martin. *Diets to Help Diabetics,* Thorsons Sterling, England, 1988.

Cavaiani, Mabel. *The High Fiber Cookbook for Diabetics,* Putnam Publishing Group, 1987.

———. *The New Diabetic Cookbook,* Contemporary Books, 1984.

Cleveland Clinic Foundation and the Department of Nutrition Staff, ed. Pat Ellis. *Cleveland Clinic Foundation Creative Cooking for Renal Diabetic Diets,* Senay Publishers, 1987.

Finsand, Mary J. *Diabetic Cakes, Pies and Other Scrumptious Desserts,* Sterling Press, 1988.

Middleton, Catherine, and Mary Abbott Hess. *The Art of Cooking for the Diabetic,* Contemporary Books, 1978.

Nutrition of the Diabetic Child: Proceedings of the Fourth Beilinson Symposium, May 21–24, 1978, S. Karger Publisher, 1980.

Wedman, Betty. *The American Diabetes Association Holiday Cookbook,* American Diabetes Association, 1986.

BOOKS DEALING WITH THE MANAGEMENT OF DIABETES

Ahuja, M. M. *Practice of Diabetes Mellitus,* Vikas Press, Vikas, India.

Anderson, James W. *Diabetes: A New Guide to Healthy Living,* Warner Books, 1983.

Arasham, Gary, and Ernest Lowe. *Diabetes: A Guide to Living Well,* DCI Publishing, 1988.

Berg, Krif E. *The Diabetic's Guide to Health and Fitness,* Human Kinetics Publishing, 1986.

Bernstein, Richard K. *Food for Diabetes: The Glucograph Method for Normalizing Blood Sugars,* Jeremy P. Tarcher, 1984.

Biermann, June, and Barbara Toohey. *The Diabetic's Total Health Book*, Jeremy P. Tarcher, 1988.

Boucher, B. J., and Ian S. Raw. *Diabetes Mellitus: Laboratory Tests and Self Monitoring*, Wolfe Medical Books, England, 1988.

Brabnin, Boris, ed. *Molecular and Cellular Biology of Diabetes Mellitus*, vols. 1–3, AR List Publisher, 1988.

Caditz, Judith. *Diabetes, Visual Impairment and Group Support: A Guide Book*, Center for the Partially Sighted, 1989.

Covelli, Pasquale, and Melvin Wiedman. *Diabetes: Current Research and Future Directions in Management and Cure*, McFarland and Company, 1988.

Creutzfeldt, W. *Acarbose for the Treatment of Diabetes Mellitus*, Springer-Verlag, 1988.

Developing Programs to Control and Prevent Diabetes: Analysis of the Problem, LBJ School of Public Affairs, 1982.

Ellenberg, Max, and Harold Rifkin, eds. *Diabetes: Theory and Practice*, 3rd and 4th eds., Prentice Hall, 1983, 1988.

Franz, Marion J. *Diabetes and Exercise: A Complete Guide for People with Diabetes or Other Chronic Health Problems*, DCI Publishing, 1990.

———. *Diabetes and Alcohol*, DCI Publishing, 1983.

Garell, Dale C., and Soloman H. Snyder. *Diabetes*, Chelsea House Publishing, 1989.

Goren, Joseph H., ed. *Insulin Action in Diabetes*, Raven Press, 1988.

Juliano, Joseph. *When Diabetes Complicates Your Life*, Chronimed DCI Publishing, 1993.

Kozak, George P. *Management of Diabetic Foot Problems*, Saunders Publishing, 1984.

Mimura, T. *Diabetes Mellitus in East Asia: Proceedings of the First China-Japan Symposium on Diabetes Mellitus*, Beijing, China, May 1988.

Selected Periodicals on Diabetes

Diabetes Forecast
Monthly magazine for diabetics published by the ADA.
The American Diabetes Association, Inc.
1660 Duke Street
Alexandria, VA 22314
Phone: 800-232-3472

Diabetes Quarterly Newsletter
Information-packed newsletter for nonmembers of the ADA.
The American Diabetes Association, Inc.
1660 Duke Street
Alexandria, VA 22314
Phone: 800-232-3472

Diabetes Interview
Informative newspaper format with topics of interest to those with
   diabetes.
3715 Balboa Street
San Francisco, CA 94121
Phone: 415-387-4002

Diabetes Self Management
Nice bimonthly publication dedicated to helping improve techniques
   in diabetes management.
P.O. Box 52890
Boulder, CO 80322
Phone: 800-234-0923

The Diabetic Reader
Excellent semiannual newsletter for the diabetic.
Barbara Toohey and June Biermann, editors
5623 Matilija Avenue
Van Nuys, CA 91401
Phone: 818-780-1308

The Diabetic Traveler
Informative monthly newsletter dedicated to the diabetic traveler.
Maury Rosenbaum, editor
P.O. Box 8223 RW
Stamford, CT 06905
Phone: 203-327-5832

The Juvenile Diabetes Foundation
Informative monthly journal that includes the latest research on
   diabetes.
432 Park Avenue South
New York, NY 10016
Phone: 800-533-2873

The Voice of the Diabetic
Quarterly publication for visually impaired and blind diabetics pre-
   pared in print and audiocassette format by the Diabetics Division
   of the National Federation of the Blind.
Ed Bryant, editor
811 Cherry Street, Suite 309
Columbia, MO 65201
Phone: 314-875-8911

COMPUTER SOFTWARE

Nutrition software is a three-program, three-disk set that computes your ideal weight, recommends a daily calorie level, and creates a daily menu plan for special needs such as diabetes, hypertension, and pregnancy. The program includes an exercise plan that calculates calories and weight loss from exercise. It monitors calories, protein, carbohydrates, fats, and cholesterol, and recommends less-caloric substitute foods from a database of 3,500 foods, including fast foods and frozen dinners.
Ohio Distinctive Software
4588 Kenney Road
Columbus, OH 43220
Phone: 614-459-0453

GOVERNMENT PUBLICATIONS

The Agriculture Handbook, Composition of Foods, Raw, Processed and Prepared, Superintendent of Documents, U.S. Government Printing Office, Washington, D.C. 20402

REFERENCES USED IN THIS BOOK

"The American Diabetes Association, Policy Statement on Artificial Sweeteners," *Diabetes Care,* page 526, volume 10, 1987.
"Nutritional Recommendations and Principles for Individuals with Diabetes Mellitus," *Diabetes Care,* volume 10, pages 126–32, 1987. Originally approved March 1987; reviewed October 1987 and October 1989.

"Oat Bran: Some Like It Hot," *University of California Wellness Letter,* 1990.

"Report on Soluble Fiber to the NANCI Corporation," Tulsa, Oklahoma, a lecture by James S. Logan, M.D., 1991.

Simms, Dorothea F., ed. *Diabetes: Reach for Health and Freedom,* page 28, C.V. Mosby, 1980.

"Use of Noncaloric Sweeteners," *Diabetes Care,* page 30, volume 16, supplement 2, May 1993.

Subject Index

Acesulfame-potassium (acesulfame-K), 46
Adolescents:
  maintaining normal growth rate in, 15
  young persons' parties and, 19–22
Air travel, 34–36
Alcohol, 14, 69
  cocktail parties and, 16–17, 18
  insulin reactions and, 17
American Academy of Pediatrics, 12
American Cancer Society, 8
American Diabetes Association, 6, 11, 47, 66, 70, 89
American Diabetes Association Diabetic Exchange Lists, 6, 365–85
  fat list, 380–82
  foods for occasional use, 385
  free foods, 382–84
  fruit list, 376–78
  general information about, 365–66
  meat list, 370–74
  milk list, 378–80
  starch/bread list, 367–70
  vegetable list, 375
American Dietetic Association, 6, 70
American Heart Association, 8, 12, 25, 70
Amoebic dysentery, 36
Appetizers, at cocktail parties, 17–18, 19
Arteriosclerosis (hardening of the arteries), 8, 53, 54
Artificial sweeteners, 41, 45–48, 383
  acesulfame-K, 46
  aspartame, 45–46
  hunger increase ascribed to, 47–48
  saccharin, 45, 47
Aspartame, 45–46

Atherosclerosis (clogged arteries), 8, 53, 54

Beans, dried, 67, 68
    exchange list for, 368
Beef, exchange list for, 372, 373, 374
Beer, 17
Beets, 75
Beverages:
    alcoholic, 14, 16–17, 18, 69
    free foods, 382
    fruit juices, 21, 30–31, 33, 34, 36, 78–81, 378
    nutrition, with fiber, 62–65
    soft drinks, 21, 34, 78–79
    vegetable juices, 78–81
Bile, 57
Birthday parties, 19–22
Blood cholesterol, 53, 58
    fiber and, 56, 57
Blood glucose, 12, 14, 52
    fiber intake and, 55–56
    fruit and, 74–75
    holiday food and, 29–30
    late-night snacks and, 38–39
    mealtime schedule and, 4, 15
    monitoring of, 42, 87–88
    normal level of, 42
    sugar alcohols and, 45
    weight gain and, 9
    see also Insulin reactions
Blood glucose meters, 49, 52
    technological advances in, 89–90
Blood lipids, 12, 14, 53
Bourbon, 17
Bread:
    exchange list for, 368–69

as fiber source, 60–61
Brown sugar, 43

Cake, 21–22
Calcium supplements, 14
Caloric intake, 12, 67
Candies, insulin reactions and, 34
Carbohydrates, 12–13
    complex, 67, 68
    simple, 68
Cardiovascular disease, 8, 15, 53, 54, 58, 70
Carrots, 75
Car trips, 32–34
Catsup, 20, 26
Cereals:
    exchange list for, 367–68
    as fiber source, 59–60
    sweeteners in, 48
Cheese, exchange list for, 372, 373, 374
Children:
    maintaining normal growth rate in, 15
    young persons' parties and, 19–22
Cholesterol intake, 13, 67
Cholesterol level, 53, 58
    fiber and, 56, 57
Citrucel, 58, 61–62
Cocktail parties, 16–19
Colon cancer, 56
Comas, hypoglycemic, 17
Complex carbohydrates, 67, 68
Compliance, 88
Computer software, on nutrition, 393

Condiments, 20, 26
  as free foods, 384
Confectioners' sugar, 43, 68
Convenience foods, 69
Corn sugar, 43
Corn syrup, 43
Crackers:
  exchange list for, 369
  as fiber source, 61
Cranberry juice, 81

Dairy products. *See* Milk
Desserts, 49–51
  fruit as, 76
  newly diagnosed Type II diabetes
    and, 50–51
  occasional enjoyment of, 49–50,
    51
Dextrin, 44
Dextrose, 42, 47
Diabetes:
  books dealing with management
    of, 389–90
  diabetic's knowledge about, 88–
    89
  incidence of, 53–54
  long-term complications of, 10–
    11, 14–15, 52–53
  magazines and newsletters on,
    391–92
  management of, 9–10, 14–15, 87–
    88; *see also* Diabetic diet
  number of people suffering from, 2
  spiritual aspects of, 90
  support role of family and friends
    and, 82–86
  technological advances in
    treatment of, 89–90

Diabetes Care, 11–12
Diabetes Forecast, 391
Diabetes Interview, 391
Diabetes Quarterly Newsletter, 391
Diabetes Self Management, 392
Diabetic diet:
  alcohol in, 14, 16–17, 18, 69
  books dealing with, 388–89
  caloric intake in, 12, 67
  carbohydrates in, 12–13, 67, 68
  cholesterol in, 13, 67
  desserts in, 49–51
  exchange lists and, 6, 365–85
  fats in, 3, 8, 12, 13, 26, 67, 71
  fiber in, 13, 52–65, 68–69
  fresh vegetables and salads in,
    70–73
  fruit and fruit sugar in, 74–77
  as healthy diet, 8, 85
  holiday food and, 28–31
  importance of, 6–15
  late-night snacks in, 38–40
  nutritional guidelines for, 66–69
  party food and drink and, 16–22
  positive attitudinal approach to,
    xv-xvi, 22, 90
  protein in, 3, 9, 13, 71
  restaurant food and, 23–27
  salt in, 14, 69
  sweeteners in, 8, 13, 41–48, 68
  thirty years ago, 7–8
  travel and, 32–37
  variety and balance in, 66–67
  vegetable and fruit juices in, 78–
    81
  vitamins and minerals in, 14
  weight control and, 15, 67
Diabetic Reader, The, 391
Diabetic Traveler, The, 392

Diarrhea, travel and, 36
Diet. *See* Diabetic diet
Digestion, 57
Digestive diseases, 54
Dips, 21
Drinks. *See* Beverages
Driving, energy consumption and, 33

Eggs, 67
  raw or lightly cooked, 387
Energy expenditure, insulin reactions and, 32–34
Equal, 45
Exchange lists. *See* American Diabetes Association Diabetic Exchange Lists
Exercise, 9, 37, 67, 87–88
Eyes, retinopathy and, 15, 53

Family, support provided by, 82–83, 85–86
Fast foods, 25–26, 69, 71
Fat (body), 10, 67
Fats (dietary): 3, 8, 12, 26, 71
  digestion of, 57
  exchange list for, 380–82
  exchange list for starch foods prepared with, 369–70
  recommended intake of, 13, 67
Fiber, 13, 52–65, 68–69, 366
  blood glucose and, 55–56
  diabetes incidence and, 53–54
  dietary, defined, 54
  feeling of fullness created by, 55
  fluid intake and, 58, 63
  health benefits of, 56–57, 58

nutrition drinks with, 62–65
removed from processed foods, 54
soluble vs. insoluble, 56
sources of, 59–61
sources of information on, 58–59
supplementing intake of, 58, 61–62
Fish, 67
  exchange list for, 372, 373, 374
Food and Drug Administration, U.S. (FDA), 46, 47
Food groups, 66–67
Foreign countries, travel to, 36
Free foods, 382–84
French fries, 26
Fried foods, 25–26
Friends, support provided by, 83–85
Fructose (fruit sugar), 21, 42–43, 44, 75, 77
Fruit juices, 21, 78–81
  exchange list for, 378
  insulin reactions and, 30–31, 33, 34, 36, 81
Fruits, 67, 68, 74–77
  blood glucose and, 74–75
  controlling quantity of, 75–76
  as dessert, 76
  exchange list for, 376–78
  fiber in, 54, 56, 57, 58
  as free foods, 383
Fruit sugar (fructose), 21, 42–43, 44, 75, 77

Game, exchange list for, 372
Glucose, 42, 43, 44
  see also Blood glucose; Blood glucose meters

Grains, 68
   exchange list for, 367–68
   fiber in, 54, 56

Hamburgers, 20, 26
Hardening of arteries
      (arteriosclerosis), 8, 53, 54
Heart, 3
Heart disease, 54, 55, 67, 71
High blood pressure
      (hypertension), 14, 68
Holiday food, 28–31
   controlling quantity of, 29–30
   mealtime schedule and, 30
Honey, 43–44
Hunger:
   artificial sweeteners and, 47–48
   fiber intake and, 55
Hypercholesterolemia, 53
Hyperglycemia, 14
Hyperlipidemia, 14, 53
Hypertension (high blood
      pressure), 14, 68
Hypertriglyceridemia, 53
Hypoglycemia. *See* Insulin reactions

Ingredient lists, 48
Insulin injections, 9
   fiber intake and, 55–56
   mealtime schedule and, 4
   reducing dosage of, 9–10, 55–56
   traveling through time zones and,
      35–36
Insulin reactions (hypoglycemia),
      14
   alcoholic beverages and, 17
   energy expenditure and, 32–34

fiber intake and, 55
friends' support and, 84–85
mealtime schedule and, 30
orange juice and, 30–31, 33, 34,
      36, 81
during sleep, 38–39
sugar-containing products for,
      34, 37
Invert sugar, 44

Juice extractors, 81
Juices:
   exchange list for, 378
   fruit, 21, 30–31, 33, 34, 36, 78–
      81, 378
   vegetable, 78–81
Juvenile Diabetes Foundation, The, 392

Kidneys, 3, 13, 15, 53, 81
Konsil D, 58, 62

Lactose (milk sugar), 43
Lamb, exchange list for, 373, 374
Late-night snacks, 38–40
Legumes, 56, 67, 68
   exchange list for, 368
Lentils, exchange list for, 368
Lipids, 12, 14, 53
Liver, 3

Maltose (malt sugar), 43
Mannitol, 44–45
Maple sugar, 44
Maple syrup, 44
Mayonnaise, 20

Mealtimes:
  during holidays, 30
  scheduling of, 3–4, 15
  traveling through time zones and,
    35
Meats, 67, 70–71
  exchange list for, 370–74
  inadequately cooked, 387
  tips for, 371
Medication, 87–88
  see also Insulin injections; Oral
    antidiabetic medication
Meditation, 90
Metamucil, 58, 62
Microangiopathy, 53
Milk, 67, 68
  exchange list for, 378–80
  as late-night snack, 39
Milk sugar (lactose), 43
Minerals, 14
Molasses, 44
Mustard, 20

NANCI Lose It, 63, 64–65
National Cancer Institute, 12, 25,
    70
Neuropathy, 14
NutraSweet (aspartame), 45–46
Nutritional guidelines, 66–69
"Nutritional Recommendations and
    Principles for Individuals with
    Diabetes Mellitus," 11–12
Nutrition drinks, with fiber, 62–65
Nutrition software, 393
Nuts, 54, 67

Oat bran, 56, 57–58
  sources of, 59–61

Obesity, 14
Olives, 75
Oral antidiabetic medication, 9
  reducing need for, 50
Orange juice, 80
  insulin reactions and, 30–31, 33,
    34, 36, 81
Overeating:
  fiber intake and, 55
  travel and, 37

Party food and drink, 16–22
  adult parties and, 16–19
  alcoholic beverages, 16–17, 18
  appetizers, 17–18, 19
  plan of action for, 18, 20
  young persons' parties and, 19–
    22
Pasta, exchange list for, 367–68
Peas (dried), exchange list for, 368
Phenylketonuria (PKU), 46
Pork, exchange list for, 372, 373,
    374
Positive mindset, xv-xvi, 22, 90
Potato chips, 20–21
Poultry, 67
  exchange list for, 372, 373
Pregnancy, 15, 69
"Principles of Nutrition and
    Dietary Guidelines for
    Individuals with Diabetes
    Mellitus," 11
Processed foods, 54, 58
Protein, 3, 9, 13, 71
  in late-night snack, 39

Raw sugar, 43
Reading list, 388–94

Renal disease, 13, 15
Restaurant food, 23–27
    freedom of choice and, 24–25, 26
Retinopathy, 15, 53
Rowles, Barbara, 48

Saccharin, 45, 47
Salad dressing, 72
Salad greens, as free foods, 383
Salads, 25, 26, 70–73
Salt, 14, 69, 366
Scotch, 17
Seasonings, as free foods, 384
Seeds, 54
Shellfish, raw, safety concerns and, 386–87
Sleep, insulin reactions during, 38–39
Snacks:
    exchange list for, 369
    late-night, 38–40
Sodium (salt), 14, 69, 366
Soft drinks, 21, 34, 78–79
Sorbitol, 44–45
Sorghum, 44
Spiritual aspects of diabetes, 90
Spoonful, 46
Starches, exchange list for, 367–70
Steak tartare, 387
Stroke, 8, 54
Sucanat, 44
Sucrose, 42, 43, 44
Sugar, 8, 13, 34, 43, 68
    in alcoholic beverages, 17
    see also Blood glucose;
        Sweeteners
Sugar alcohols, 41, 44–45
Support groups, 89

Sweeteners, 8, 13, 41–48, 68
    in condiments, 20
    ingredients lists and, 48
    noncaloric, nonnutritive
        (artificial), 41, 45–48, 383
    nutritive, with chemical names,
        41, 42–43
    nutritive, with common names,
        41, 43–44
Sweet'n Low, 47
Sweet One, 46

Tequila, 17
Time zones, traveling through, 35–36
Travel, 32–37
    air, 34–36
    car, 32–34
    to foreign countries, 36
    insulin dosage and, 35–36
    mealtime schedule and, 35
    through time zones, 35–36
Travelers' diarrhea, 36
Triglycerides, 53, 55
Turbinado sugar, 43
Type I insulin-dependent diabetes, 2
    management of, 9
    traveling through time zones and,
        35–36
Type II non-insulin-dependent
        diabetes, 2
    desserts and, 50–51
    management of, 9–10

Ultra Slim Fast, 62–64
Urinary tract, 81
U.S. Dietary Guidelines, 12

Veal, exchange list for, 372, 373
Vegetable juices, 78–81
Vegetables, 25, 67, 68, 70–73
  buying and storing, 72–73
  exchange list for, 375
  fiber in, 54, 56, 57, 58
  free foods, 383
  starchy, exchange list for, 368
Vegetarian diet, 70
V-8 vegetable juice, 79–80
Vibrio infection, 386

Vitamins, 14
Vodka, 17
Voice of the Diabetic, The, 392

Weight, 9, 15, 67
  late-night snack and, 39
Whiskey, 17
Wine, 17

Xylitol, 44–45

Recipe Index

Accompaniments. *See* Condiments;
    Side dishes
Acini, Sautéed, 254–55
Acorn Squash, Stuffed, 229–30
Almond(s):
    Cranberry-Nut Bread, 318–19
    Strawberry Bread, 316–17
Ancho chili:
    Glaze, 165
    Sauce, 163–65
Appetizers, 95–110
    Ceviche, 299–300
    Hot Tofu Salad, 107
    Pita Crisps, 103–4
    Roasted Eggplant Dip, 102–3
    Sautéed or Grilled Ginger Tofu
        with Teriyaki Sauce, 104–6
    Spinach Dip, 101
    Texas Pesto, 98–99
    Vegetable Hummus, 97–98
    Vegetable Rotella, 108–10
    Yogurt and Cucumber Dip,
        100

Apple(s):
    Brussels Sprout Sauté with
        Onions and, 217–18
    Caraway, and Cabbage Salad,
        189–90
    Pancake, German, 118–20
    Slices, Spicy, 308–9
    and Sweet Potato Scallop, 236–37
Applesauce, 307
    Cake, Spicy, 341–42
    Soufflé, 346–47
Artichokes, Tofu Chicken Casserole
        with Mushrooms and, 276–78
Asian dishes:
    Carrot and Sweet Potato Soup,
        150–51
    Sautéed or Grilled Ginger Tofu
        with Teriyaki Sauce, 104–6
    Spicy Chilled Soba Noodles,
        258–60
    Steamed or Microwaved Ginger
        Fish with Soy, 285–86
    Thai Tofu Salad, 207–8

Baked:
  Chiles Rellenos, 302–4
  Corn, 220–21
  Flounder with Ginger and
    Oranges, 288–89
  Herbal Rice with Pine Nuts,
    246–47
  Spiced Fish, 283–84
Banana:
  Dynamite, 76
  and Strawberry Yogurt Pie, 324–
    25
Barley:
  Cucumber, and Tomato Salad
    with Yogurt Dressing, 196–97
  Mushroom Pilaf, 231–32
Basil, in Texas Pesto, 98–99
Bean curd. *See* Tofu
Beans, Green, with Mustard and
    Ginger, 223–24
Beef:
  Broth, 135–36
  Red Pepper Steak, 281–82
Beet(s):
  Chilled Blender Borscht, 144–
    45
  -Top Borscht, 141–43
Blackberry Pudding with Lemon
    Wine Sauce, 350–51
Blueberry Pudding with Lemon
    Wine Sauce, 350–51
Borscht:
  Beet-Top, 141–43
  Chilled Blender, 144–45
Bow Tie Pasta with Roasted Red,
    Yellow, and Green Bell
    Peppers, 255–56
Braised Salmon and Halibut
    Steaks, 292–93

Bread(s):
  Cranberry-Nut, 318–19
  crumbs, 275
  Sourdough, Pudding, 352–53
  Strawberry-Almond, 316–17
Breakfast fare, 111–23
  Basic Omelet Recipe and
    Fillings, 120–23
  Cottage Cheese Muffins, 113–14
  Cottage Cheese Pancakes, 115–18
  Cranberry Acerola Super Shake,
    65
  German Apple Pancake, 118–20
Broccoli:
  Lemon, 215–16
  Winter Green Soup, 140–41
Broiled:
  Chicken Tarragon with Wine,
    269–70
  Chicken with Vegetable
    Vinaigrette, 272–74
  Fish with Tomatoes, Garlic, and
    Chilies, 287–88
  Tuna with Mango-Papaya
    Relish, 290–91
Broths:
  Beef, 135–36
  Chicken, 133–34
  Garlic, 132–33
  Potato Peel, 129–31
  Vegetable, 128–29
Brunch fare:
  Orange, Grapefruit, and
    Raspberry Terrine, 356–59
  see also Breakfast fare
Brussels Sprout Sauté with Apples
    and Onions, 217–18
Bulgur Wheat Salad (Tabbouleh),
    203–4

Cabbage:
  Caraway, and Apple Salad, 189–90
  red, in Spicy Red Coleslaw, 186–87
  red, potato, and carrot omelet filling, 123
  Salad, 185
Cakes:
  Cardamom Cream, 334–35
  Carrot, 343–44
  Chocolate Fudge, with Chocolate Icing, 339–40
  Spicy Applesauce, 341–42
Caraway, Cabbage, and Apple Salad, 189–90
Cardamom Cream Cake, 334–35
Cardinal Peaches with Raspberries, 311–12
Carrot(s):
  Cake, 343–44
  Lemon, 216
  potato, and red cabbage omelet filling, 123
  Salad, Curried, 188
  and Sweet Potato Soup, 150–51
Casseroles:
  Baked Chiles Rellenos, 302–4
  Herbed Soybean, 221–23
  Tofu Chicken, with Mushrooms and Artichokes, 276–78
Cauliflower:
  Lemon, 216
  and Mixed Pepper Salad, 190–92
Ceviche, 299–300
"Chantilly," Sweet Potato and Fresh Peach, 314–16

Cheese:
  Cottage, Muffins, 113–14
  Cottage, Pancakes, 115–18
  Feta, Vegetable Salad with, 200–201
  Parmesan, Eggplant, 226–27
  -and-Tofu-Stuffed Jumbo Shells, 301–2
Chicken:
  Breasts, Honeyed, 278–80
  Breasts, Lime, 265–66
  Breasts, Roasted, 266–67
  Broiled, with Tarragon and Wine, 269–70
  Broth, 133–34
  Greek, 268–69
  Grilled or Broiled, with Vegetable Vinaigrette, 272–74
  marinating, 263
  Mulligatawny Soup (Stew), 157–59
  Provençale, 274–76
  Salad, Crunchy, 210–11
  Salad, Southwestern, 209–10
  Salad, Thai, 207–8
  southwestern omelet filling, 122
  Spiced, with Spinach, 271–72
  Tofu Casserole with Mushrooms and Artichokes, 276–78
Chick-peas, in Vegetable Hummus, 97–98
Chiles Rellenos, Baked, 302–4
Chili(es):
  Ancho, Glaze, 165
  Ancho, Sauce, 163–65
  Broiled Fish with Tomatoes, Garlic and, 287–88
Chilled Blender Borscht, 144–45

Chocolate:
  Crepes, 359–61
  Fudge Cake with Chocolate
    Icing, 339–40
  Pudding, Steamed, 337–38
Chutneys:
  Cranberry, 177–78
  Spicy Pineapple, 175–76
Cilantro, in Texas Pesto, 98–99
Cioppino, Northwest, 156–57
Clams, Linguini with, 257–58
Coconut and Lime Mousse, 353–55
Coleslaw, Spicy Red, 186–87
Compote, Fruit, 312–14
Condiments, 161–82
  Cranberry Chutney, 177–78
  Fresh Cranberry, Tangerine, and
    Lime Relish, 178–79
  Mango-Papaya Relish, 290–91
  Pear Relish, 179–80
  Pickled Bell Peppers, 181–82
  Spicy Pineapple Chutney, 175–
    76
  Texas Pesto, 98–99
  see also Sauces
Corn:
  Baked, 220–21
  "Creamed," 218–19
  Fresh, and Wild Rice Sauté,
    251–52
  and Tortilla Soup, Spicy, 151–53
Cottage cheese:
  Muffins, 113–14
  Pancakes, 115–18
Cranberry:
  Acerola Super Shake, 65
  Chutney, 177–78
  Nut Bread, 318–19
  and Rice Stuffing, 248–49

Salsa, 169
Sauce, 167–68
Tangerine, and Lime Relish, 178–
  79
Cream, Vanilla Custard, 363–64
"Creamed" Corn, 218–19
Creamed Potatoes, Skillet, 237–38
Cream Puffs, 361–63
Creole dishes:
  Rice Custard, 344–45
  Wild Rice and Shrimp, 252–53
Crepes, Chocolate, 359–61
Crunchy Chicken Salad, 210–11
Cucumber:
  Barley, and Tomato Salad with
    Yogurt Dressing, 196–97
  Salad, Dilled, 193–94
  Salad, Persian, 195
  and Yogurt Dip, 100
Cumin, New Potatoes with
  Turmeric and, 235–36
Curry(ied):
  Carrot Salad, 188
  Potatoes, 239–40
Custard:
  Creole Rice, 344–45
  "Slipped," Pie, 325–27
  Vanilla, Cream, 363–64

Desserts, 305–64
  Applesauce, 307
  Banana Dynamite, 76
  Blueberry or Blackberry
    Pudding with Lemon Wine
    Sauce, 350–51
  Cardamom Cream Cake, 334–35
  Cardinal Peaches with
    Raspberries, 311–12

Carrot Cake, 343–44
Chocolate Crepes, 359–61
Chocolate Fudge Cake with
    Chocolate Icing, 339–40
Cranberry-Nut Bread, 318–19
Cream Puffs, 361–63
Creole Rice Custard, 344–45
Fresh Fruit Soufflé, 346–47
Fresh Rhubarb and Strawberry
    Pie, 330–31
Fruit Compote, 312–14
German Apple Pancake, 118–20
Lime and Coconut Mousse, 353–
    55
Mixed Fruit Pie, 332–33
Orange, Grapefruit, and
    Raspberry Terrine, 356–59
Pears Poached in Red Wine,
    309–10
prune puree as substitute for fat
    in, 336–37
Rice Pudding, 348–49
"Slipped" Custard Pie, 325–27
Sourdough Bread Pudding, 352–
    53
Spicy Applesauce Cake, 341–42
Spicy Apple Slices, 308–9
Steamed Chocolate Pudding,
    337–38
Strawberry-Almond Bread, 316–
    17
Strawberry and Banana Yogurt
    Pie, 324–25
Sweet Potato and Fresh Peach
    "Chantilly," 314–16
Sweet Potato Pie, 328–29
Vanilla Custard Cream, 363–
    64
Dilled Cucumber Salad, 193–94

Dips:
    Pita Crisps for, 103–4
    Roasted Eggplant, 102–3
    Spinach, 101
    Texas Pesto, 98–99
    Tomatillo Sauce (Salsa Verdes),
        165–67
    Vegetable Hummus, 97–98
    Yogurt and Cucumber, 100

Eggplant:
    Asian, Sautéed with Snow Peas,
        227–28
    Parmesan, 226
    Roasted, Dip, 102–3
    Vegetable Rotella, 108–10
Eggs:
    Baked Chiles Rellenos, 302–4
    Basic Omelet Recipe and
        Fillings, 120–23
    separating, 120
Enchilada Sauce, 165
Entrées, 261–304
    Baked Chiles Rellenos, 302–4
    Baked Flounder with Ginger and
        Oranges, 288–89
    Bow Tie Pasta with Roasted
        Red, Yellow, and Green Bell
        Peppers, 255–56
    Braised Salmon and Halibut
        Steaks, 292–93
    Broiled Chicken Tarragon with
        Wine, 269–70
    Broiled Fish with Tomatoes,
        Garlic, and Chilies, 287–88
    Ceviche, 299–300
    Chicken Provençale, 274–76
    Crunchy Chicken Salad, 210–11

Entrées (*cont'd*)
Eggplant Parmesan, 226–27
Greek Chicken, 268–69
Grilled or Broiled Chicken with
  Vegetable Vinaigrette, 272–74
Grilled or Broiled Tuna with
  Mango-Papaya Relish, 290–
  91
Halibut Kebabs, 295–97
Herbed Soybean Casserole, 221–
  23
Honeyed Chicken Breasts, 278–
  80
Lime Chicken Breasts, 265–66
Linguine with Clams, 257–58
Poached Salmon, 282–83
Portuguese Fish Stew, 297–98
Red Pepper Steak, 281–82
Roasted Chicken Breasts, 266–
  67
Sautéed Asian Eggplant with
  Snow Peas, 227–28
soup as, 127
Southwestern Chicken Salad,
  209–10
Spiced Baked Fish, 283–84
Spiced Chicken with Spinach,
  271–72
Steamed or Microwaved Ginger
  Fish with Soy, 285–86
Stir-fried Shrimp with Peas and
  Water Chestnuts, 293–95
Stuffed Acorn Squash, 229–30
Thai Tofu Salad, 207–8
Tofu-and-Cheese-Stuffed Jumbo
  Shells, 301–2
Tofu Chicken Casserole with
  Mushrooms and Artichokes,
  276–78

Wild Rice and Shrimp Creole,
  252–53

Fat, prune puree as substitute for,
  336–37
Feta Cheese, Vegetable Salad with,
  200–201
Fish:
  Baked Flounder with Ginger and
    Oranges, 288–89
  Braised Salmon and Halibut
    Steaks, 292–93
  Broiled, with Tomatoes, Garlic,
    and Chilies, 287–88
  Ceviche, 299–300
  Grilled or Broiled Tuna with
    Mango-Papaya Relish, 290–91
  Halibut Kebabs, 295–97
  marinating, 263
  Northwest Cioppino, 156–57
  Poached Salmon, 282–83
  Soup, Lime-Tarragon French
    (Pot- au-Feu), 153–55
  Spiced Baked, 283–84
  Steamed or Microwaved Ginger,
    with Soy, 285–86
  Stew, Portuguese, 297–98
  see also Shellfish
Flounder Baked with Ginger and
  Oranges, 288–89
French dishes:
  Chicken Provençale, 274–76
  Lime-Tarragon Fish Soup (Pot-
    au-Feu), 153–55
Fresh Rhubarb and Strawberry
  Pie, 330–31
Fritters, Spicy Sweet Potato, 241–
  42

Fruit:
    Compote, 312–14
    Fresh, Soufflé, 346–47
    Mixed, Pie, 332–33
    see also specific fruits
Fudge, Chocolate, Cake with
    Chocolate Icing, 339–40

Garlic:
    Broiled Fish with Tomatoes,
        Chilies and, 287–88
    Broth, 132–33
German Apple Pancake, 118–
    20
Ginger:
    Baked Flounder with Oranges
        and, 288–89
    Fish with Soy, Steamed or
        Microwaved, 285–86
    Green Beans with Mustard and,
        223–24
    Tofu, Sautéed or Grilled, with
        Teriyaki Sauce, 104–6
Grapefruit, Orange, and Raspberry
    Terrine, 356–59
Greek dishes:
    Chicken, 268–69
    Salad, 199
Green Beans with Mustard and
    Ginger, 223–24
Green Soup, Winter, 140–41
Grilled:
    Chicken with Vegetable
        Vinaigrette, 272–74
    Ginger Tofu with Teriyaki Sauce,
        104–6
    Tuna with Mango-Papaya
        Relish, 290–91

Halibut:
    Kebabs, 295–97
    and Salmon Steaks, Braised,
        292–93
Herbal Baked Rice with Pine Nuts,
    246–47
Herbed Soybean Casserole, 221–
    23
Honeyed Chicken Breasts, 278–80
Hot Tofu Salad, 107
Hummus, Vegetable, 97–98

Icing, Chocolate, 339–40
Indian dishes:
    Mulligatawny Soup (Stew), 157–
        59
    Spicy Pineapple Chutney, 175–
        76
Italian dishes:
    Eggplant Parmesan, 226–27
    Jiffy Marinara Sauce, 173–
        74
    Marinara Sauce, 171–73
    Risotto with Spinach, 249–50

Kebabs, Halibut, 295–97

Lemon:
    Broccoli, 215–16
    Carrots, 216
    Cauliflower, 216
    Wine Sauce, Blueberry or
        Blackberry Pudding with,
        350–51
    Zucchini or Yellow Crookneck
        Squash, 216

Lentil(s):
  Mulligatawny Soup (Stew), 157–
    59
  Salad, 202–3
Lime:
  Chicken Breasts, 265–66
  and Coconut Mousse, 353–55
  Fresh Cranberry, and Tangerine
    Relish, 178–79
  Rice, 245
  Tarragon French Fish Soup
    (Pot-au-Feu), 153–55
Linguini with Clams, 257–58
Lyonnaise Potatoes, 240–41

Mango-Papaya Relish, 290–
  91
Marinara Sauce, 171–73
  Jiffy, 173–74
Marinating, 263
Meat:
  marinating, 263
  see also Beef
Mediterranean Salad, 197–98
Meringue Piecrust, 322–23
Mexican and southwestern dishes:
  Ancho Chili Sauce, 163–65
  Baked Chiles Rellenos, 302–4
  Ceviche, 299–300
  omelet filling, 122
  Pico de Gallo Salsa, 170–71
  Southwestern Chicken Salad,
    209–10
  Texas Pesto, 98–99
  Tomatillo Sauce (*Salsa Verdes*),
    165–67
Microwaved Ginger Fish with Soy,
  285–86

Minestrone, 148–49
Mousse, Lime and Coconut, 353–
  55
Muffins, Cottage Cheese, 113–14
Mulligatawny Soup (Stew), 157–
  59
Mushroom(s):
  Barley Pilaf, 231–32
  and spinach omelet filling, 122
  Tofu Chicken Casserole with
    Artichokes and, 276–78
Mustard, Green Beans with Ginger
  and, 223–24

Noodle(s):
  Soba, Spicy Chilled, 258–60
  Soup, Simple, 137–38
  see also Pasta
Northwest Cioppino, 156–57
Nut Bread, Cranberry, 318–19

Omelet Recipe and Fillings, Basic,
  120–23
Onion(s):
  Brussels Sprout Sauté with
    Apples and, 217–18
  Mediterranean Salad, 197–98
  Red, Spinach, and Tomato Salad,
    192–93
  Soup, 145–47
Orange(s):
  Baked Flounder with Ginger
    and, 288–89
  Grapefruit, and Raspberry
    Terrine, 356–59
  Mediterranean Salad, 197–
    98

Pancake(s):
    Cottage Cheese, 115–18
    German Apple, 118–20
Papaya-Mango Relish, 290–91
Parmesan, Eggplant, 226
Pasta:
    Bow Tie, with Roasted Red,
        Yellow, and Green Bell
        Peppers, 255–56
    Chicken Provençale, 274–76
    Linguini with Clams, 257–58
    Sautéed Acini, 254–55
    Tofu-and-Cheese-Stuffed Jumbo
        Shells, 301–2
    Vegetable Rotella, 108–10
    Vegetable Salad, Tomatoes
        Stuffed with, 205–6
    see also Noodle(s)
Peach(es):
    Cardinal, with Raspberries, 311–
        12
    Fresh, and Sweet Potato
        "Chantilly," 314–16
Pear(s):
    Poached in Red Wine, 309–10
    Relish, 179–80
Peas:
    Stir-fried Shrimp with Water
        Chestnuts and, 293–95
    Winter Green Soup, 140–41
Pepper(s) (bell):
    Mixed, and Cauliflower Salad,
        190–92
    omelet filling, 122
    Pickled, 181–82
    Red, Steak, 281–82
    Roasted Red, Yellow, and Green,
        Bow Tie Pasta with, 255–56
    roasting, 264

Persian Cucumber Salad, 195
Pesto, Texas, 98–99
Pickled Bell Peppers, 181–82
Pico de Gallo Salsa, 170–71
Piecrusts:
    Basic Single, 319–22
    Meringue, 322–23
Pies:
    Banana and Strawberry Yogurt,
        324–25
    Fresh Rhubarb and Strawberry,
        330–31
    Mixed Fruit, 332–33
    "Slipped" Custard, 325–27
    Sweet Potato, 328–29
Pilaf, Barley-Mushroom, 231–32
Pineapple Chutney, Spicy, 175–76
Pine Nuts, Herbal Baked Rice
        with, 246–47
Pita Crisps, 103–4
Poached:
    Pears, in Red Wine, 309–10
    Salmon, 282–83
Portuguese Fish Stew, 297–98
Potato(es):
    carrot, and red cabbage omelet
        filling, 123
    Curried, 239–40
    Lyonnaise, 240–41
    New, Roasted, 234
    New, with Turmeric and Cumin,
        235–36
    Peel Broth, 129–31
    Roasted Sliced, 233–34
    Skillet Creamed, 237–38
    see also Sweet potato(es)
Pot-au-Feu (Lime-Tarragon French
        Fish Soup), 153–55
Provençale, Chicken, 274–76

Prune Puree, 336–37
Puddings:
  Blueberry or Blackberry, with
    Lemon Wine Sauce, 350–51
  Rice, 348–49
  Sourdough Bread, 352–53
  Steamed Chocolate, 337–38

Radishes, in Spicy Red Coleslaw,
  186–87
Raspberry(ies):
  Cardinal Peaches with, 311–12
  Orange, and Grapefruit Terrine,
    356–59
Relishes:
  Fresh Cranberry, Tangerine, and
    Lime, 178–79
  Mango-Papaya, 290–91
  Pear, 179–80
  see also Chutneys
Rhubarb and Strawberry Pie, 330–
  31
Rice:
  and Cranberry Stuffing, 248–
    49
  Custard, Creole, 344–45
  Herbal Baked, with Pine Nuts,
    246–47
  Lime, 245
  Powder, Roasted, 208
  Pudding, 348–49
  Risotto with Spinach, 249–50
  Stuffed Acorn Squash, 229–30
  see also Wild rice
Risotto with Spinach, 249–50
Roasted:
  Chicken Breasts, 266–67
  Eggplant Dip, 102–3

Red, Yellow, and Green Bell
  Peppers, Bow Tie Pasta with,
  255–56
Rice Powder, 208
Sliced Potatoes, 233–34
Roasting peppers, 264
Rotella, Vegetable, 108–10

Salad dressings, 187, 189, 191, 200–
  201
  Tarragon, 206
Salads, 183–211
  Barley, Cucumber, and Tomato,
    with Yogurt Dressing, 196–97
  Bulgur Wheat (Tabbouleh),
    203–4
  Cabbage, 185
  Caraway, Cabbage, and Apple,
    189–90
  Cauliflower and Mixed Pepper,
    190–92
  Crunchy Chicken, 210–11
  Curried Carrot, 188
  Dilled Cucumber, 193–94
  Greek, 199
  Hot Tofu, 107
  Lentil, 202–3
  Mediterranean, 197–98
  Persian Cucumber, 195
  Southwestern Chicken, 209–10
  Spicy Red Coleslaw, 186–87
  Spinach, Tomato, and Red
    Onion, 192–93
  Thai Tofu, 207–8
  Tomatoes Stuffed with Vegetable
    Pasta, 205–6
  Vegetable, with Feta Cheese,
    200–201

Salmon:
   and Halibut Steaks, Braised,
      292–93
   Poached, 282–83
Salsa:
   Cranberry, 169
   Pico de Gallo, 170–71
   Verdes (Tomatillo Sauce), 165–
      67
Sauces:
   Ancho Chili, 163–65
   Cranberry, 167–68
   Cranberry Salsa, 169
   Enchilada, 165
   Jiffy Marinara, 173–74
   Marinara, 171–73
   Pico de Gallo Salsa, 170–71
   Teriyaki, 104–5, 106
   Tomatillo (*Salsa Verdes*), 165–67
   Vanilla Custard Cream, 363–64
Sauté(ed):
   Acini, 254–55
   Asian Eggplant with Snow Peas,
      227–28
   Brussels Sprout, with Apples and
      Onions, 217–18
   Fresh Corn and Wild Rice, 251–
      52
   Ginger Tofu with Teriyaki Sauce,
      104–6
   Spinach, 225
Scallops, in Northwest Cioppino,
   156–57
Shake, Cranberry Acerola Super,
   65
Shellfish:
   Ceviche, 299–300
   Linguini with Clams, 257–58
   Northwest Cioppino, 156–57

Stir-fried Shrimp with Peas and
   Water Chestnuts, 293–95
Wild Rice and Shrimp Creole,
   252–53
Shells, Jumbo, Tofu-and-Cheese-
   Stuffed, 301–2
Shrimp:
   Northwest Cioppino, 156–57
   Stir-fried with Peas and Water
      Chestnuts, 293–95
   and Wild Rice Creole, 252–53
Side dishes:
   Applesauce, 307
   Baked Corn, 220–21
   Barley, Cucumber, and Tomato
      Salad with Yogurt Dressing,
      196–97
   Barley-Mushroom Pilaf, 231–
      32
   Brussels Sprout Sauté with
      Apples and Onions, 217–18
   Bulgur Wheat Salad
      (Tabbouleh), 203–4
   Cabbage Salad, 185
   Caraway, Cabbage, and Apple
      Salad, 189–90
   Cauliflower and Mixed Pepper
      Salad, 190–92
   "Creamed" Corn, 218–19
   Curried Carrot Salad, 188
   Curried Potatoes, 239–40
   Dilled Cucumber Salad, 193–94
   Eggplant Parmesan, 226
   Fresh Corn and Wild Rice Sauté,
      251–52
   Fruit Compote, 312–14
   Greek Salad, 199
   Green Beans with Mustard and
      Ginger, 223–24

Side dishes (*cont'd*)
  Herbed Soybean Casserole, 221–23
  Lemon Broccoli, 215–16
  Lentil Salad, 202–3
  Lyonnaise Potatoes, 240–41
  Mediterranean Salad, 197–98
  New Potatoes with Turmeric and Cumin, 235–36
  Persian Cucumber Salad, 195
  Roasted Sliced Potatoes, 233–34
  Sautéed Acini, 254–55
  Sautéed Asian Eggplant with Snow Peas, 227–28
  Skillet Creamed Potatoes, 237–38
  Spicy Chilled Soba Noodles, 258–60
  Spicy Red Coleslaw, 186–87
  Spicy Sweet Potato Fritters, 241–42
  Spinach, Tomato, and Red Onion Salad, 192–93
  Spinach Sauté, 225
  Stuffed Acorn Squash, 229–30
  Sweet Potato and Apple Scallop, 236–37
  Tomatoes Stuffed with Vegetable Pasta Salad, 205–6
  Vegetable Salad with Feta Cheese, 200–201
  see also Condiments; Rice
Skillet Creamed Potatoes, 237–38
"Slipped" Custard Pie, 325–27
Snow Peas, Sautéed Asian Eggplant with, 227–28
Soba Noodles, Spicy Chilled, 258–60
Soufflé, Fresh Fruit, 346–47

Soups, 125–59
  Beet-Top Borscht, 141–43
  Carrot and Sweet Potato, 150–51
  Chilled Blender Borscht, 144–45
  as entreé, 127
  Lime-Tarragon French Fish (Pot-au-Feu), 153–55
  Minestrone, 148–49
  Mulligatawny, 157–59
  Northwest Cioppino, 156–57
  Onion, 145–47
  Simple Noodle, 137–38
  Spicy Corn-and-Tortilla, 151–53
  Spinach, 138–39
  Winter Green, 140–41
  see also Broths
Sourdough Bread Pudding, 352–53
Southwestern dishes. *See* Mexican and southwestern dishes
Soy, Steamed or Microwaved Ginger Fish with, 285–86
Soybean Casserole, Herbed, 221–23
Spiced:
  Baked Fish, 283–84
  Chicken with Spinach, 271–72
Spicy:
  Applesauce Cake, 341–42
  Apple Slices, 308–9
  Chilled Soba Noodles, 258–60
  Corn-and-Tortilla Soup, 151–53
  Pineapple Chutney, 175–76
  Red Coleslaw, 186–87
  Sweet Potato Fritters, 241–42
Spinach:
  Dip, 101
  and mushroom omelet filling, 122
  Risotto with, 249–50
  Sauté, 225
  Soup, 138–39

Spiced Chicken with, 271–72
Tomato, and Red Onion Salad,
  192–93
Winter Green Soup, 140–41
Squash:
Acorn, Stuffed, 229–30
yellow crookneck, in Herbed
  Soybean Casserole, 221–23
Yellow Crookneck, Lemon, 216
see also Zucchini
Steak, Red Pepper, 281–82
Steamed:
Chocolate Pudding, 337–38
Ginger Fish with Soy, 285–86
Stews:
Mulligatawny, 157–59
Northwest Cioppino, 156–57
Portuguese Fish, 297–98
Wild Rice and Shrimp Creole,
  252–53
Stir-fried Shrimp with Peas and
  Water Chestnuts, 293–95
Stocks. *See* Broths
Strawberry:
Almond Bread, 316–17
and Banana Yogurt Pie, 324–25
Fresh Rhubarb and, Pie, 330–31
Stuffed Acorn Squash, 229–30
Stuffing, Rice and Cranberry, 248–49
Sweet potato(es):
and Apple Scallop, 236–37
and Carrot Soup, 150–51
and Fresh Peach "Chantilly,"
  314–16
Fritters, Spicy, 241–42
Pie, 328–29

Tabbouleh (Bulgur Wheat Salad),
  203–4

Tahini, in Vegetable Hummus, 97–98
Tangerine, Fresh Cranberry, and
  Lime Relish, 178–79
Tarragon:
Chicken with Wine, Broiled,
  269–70
Dressing, 206
Lime French Fish Soup (Pot-au-
  Feu), 153–55
Teriyaki Sauce, 104–5, 106
Terrine, Orange, Grapefruit, and
  Raspberry, 356–59
Texas Pesto, 98–99
Thai Tofu Salad, 207–8
Tofu (bean curd):
-and-Cheese-Stuffed Jumbo
  Shells, 301–2
Chicken Casserole with
  Mushrooms and Artichokes,
  276–78
marinating, 263
Salad, Hot, 107
Salad, Thai, 207–8
Sautéed or Grilled Ginger, with
  Teriyaki Sauce, 104–6
Tomatillo Sauce (*Salsa Verdes*), 165–67
Tomato(es):
Barley, and Cucumber Salad
  with Yogurt Dressing, 196–97
Broiled Fish with Garlic, Chilies
  and, 287–88
Herbed Soybean Casserole, 221–
  23
Jiffy Marinara Sauce, 173–74
Marinara Sauce, 171–73
Spinach, and Red Onion Salad,
  192–93
Stuffed with Vegetable Pasta
  Salad, 205–6

Tortilla and Corn Soup, Spicy, 151–53

Tuna, Grilled or Broiled, with Mango-Papaya Relish, 290–91

Turmeric, New Potatoes with Cumin and, 235–36

Vanilla Custard Cream, 363–64

Vegetable(s), 213–42
  Baked Corn, 220–21
  Barley-Mushroom Pilaf, 231–32
  Broth, 128–29
  Brussels Sprout Sauté with Apples and Onions, 217–18
  "Creamed" Corn, 218–19
  Curried Potatoes, 239–40
  Eggplant Parmesan, 226
  Green Beans with Mustard and Ginger, 223–24
  Grilled or Broiled Chicken with, Vinaigrette, 272–74
  Herbed Soybean Casserole, 221–23
  Hummus, 97–98
  Lemon Broccoli, 215–16
  Lyonnaise Potatoes, 240–41
  marinating, 263
  Minestrone, 148–49
  New Potatoes with Turmeric and Cumin, 235–36
  Pasta Salad, Tomatoes Stuffed with, 205–6
  Roasted Sliced Potatoes, 233–34
  Rotella, 108–10
  Salad with Feta Cheese, 200–201
  Sautéed Asian Eggplant with Snow Peas, 227–28
  Skillet Creamed Potatoes, 237–38

Spicy Sweet Potato Fritters, 241–42

Spinach Sauté, 225

Stuffed Acorn Squash, 229–30

Sweet Potato and Apple Scallop, 236–37

Water Chestnuts, Stir-fried Shrimp with Peas and, 293–95

Wild rice:
  and Fresh Corn Sauté, 251–52
  and Shrimp Creole, 252–53

Wine:
  Broiled Chicken Tarragon with, 269–70
  Lemon Sauce, Blueberry or Blackberry Pudding with, 350–51
  Red, Pears Poached in, 309–10

Winter Green Soup, 140–41

Yellow crookneck squash:
  Herbed Soybean Casserole, 221–23
  Lemon, 216

Yogurt:
  Banana and Strawberry, Pie, 324–25
  and Cucumber Dip, 100
  Dressing, Barley, Cucumber, and Tomato Salad with, 196–97

Zucchini:
  Barley-Mushroom Pilaf as stuffing for, 231
  Lemon, 216
  Winter Green Soup, 140–41